Pocket Pediatric Emergency Medicine Course for Interns

Disclaimer

Every effort has been made to ensure that the drug dosages herein are accurate and in accordance with the standards accepted at the time of publication. However, the user is advised to check the doses carefully. The author is not responsible for any error in this publication. Besides, as new research and experience broaden our knowledge, changes in treatment and drug therapy occur. Therefore, the reader is advised to read the product information included in the package of the recommended dosage and contraindications. In addition, the protocols included in the book are valid at the time of publication and are subjected to constant review.

The protocols have been specific for medical colleges, wherein the intern will handle the initial hour of resuscitation prior to the arrival of more experienced help.

Pocket Pediatric Emergency Medicine Course for Interns

Editor

Indumathy Santhanam MD DCH

Professor of Pediatrics
Head, Department of Pediatric Emergency Medicine
Institute of Child Health
Madras Medical College
Chennai, Tamil Nadu, India

"In resuscitation, perfection is not optional"
—*Peter Safer (Father of modern CPR)*

JAYPEE *The Health Sciences Publisher*
New Delhi | London | Panama

Jaypee Brothers Medical Publishers (P) Ltd

Headquarters
Jaypee Brothers Medical Publishers (P) Ltd.
4838/24, Ansari Road, Daryaganj
New Delhi 110 002, India
Phone: +91-11-43574357
Fax: +91-11-43574314
E-mail: jaypee@jaypeebrothers.com

Overseas Offices
JP Medical Ltd.
83, Victoria Street, London
SW1H 0HW (UK)
Phone: +44-20 3170 8910
Fax: +44(0)20 3008 6180
E-mail: info@jpmedpub.com

Jaypee-Highlights Medical Publishers Inc.
City of Knowledge, Bld. 235, 2nd Floor, Clayton
Panama City, Panama
Phone: +1 507-301-0496
Fax: +1 507-301-0499
E-mail: cservice@jphmedical.com

Jaypee Brothers Medical Publishers (P) Ltd.
17/1-B, Babar Road, Block-B, Shyamoli
Mohammadpur, Dhaka-1207
Bangladesh
Mobile: +08801912003485
E-mail: jaypeedhaka@gmail.com

Jaypee Brothers Medical Publishers (P) Ltd.
Bhotahity, Kathmandu, Nepal
Phone: +977-9741283608
E-mail: kathmandu@jaypeebrothers.com

Website: www.jaypeebrothers.com
Website: www.jaypeedigital.com

Pocket Pediatric Emergency Medicine Course for Interns

First Edition: 2018

ISBN: 978-93-86261-62-5

Printed at: Samrat Offset Pvt. Ltd.

Dedication

This book is dedicated to the nurses in the Pediatric Emergency Department of the Institute of Child Health, Madras Medical College, whose untiring efforts and expertise give hope to every mother, who brings her critically ill child to our threshold.

Contributors

Indumathy Santhanam MD DCH
Professor of Pediatrics
Head, Department of Pediatric Emergency Medicine, Institute of Child Health
Madras Medical College
Chennai, Tamil Nadu, India

Gundas Srininvasan DCH DNB
Fellow in Pediatric Emergency Medicine
Pediatric Emergency Service
Manipal Hospital
Bengaluru, Karnataka, India

Decision-making Triangles

J Balaji MD
Associate Professor of Pediatrics
Department of Pediatrics
Government Dharmapuri Medical College
Dharmapuri, Tamil Nadu, India

Approach to Fever in Children
Acute Gastroenteritis
Lower Respiratory Tract Infections
Typhoid Fever
Prophylaxis

T Murali MD DCH FPEM
Senior Assistant Professor
Pediatric Emergency Department
Institute of Child Health
Madras Medical College
Chennai, Tamil Nadu, India

BLS

Chandan Kumar MD FPEM
Fellow-Pediatric Emergency Medicine
Institute of Child Health
Madras Medical College
Chennai, Tamil Nadu, India

Trauma

V Poornachand MD
Postgraduate
Institute of Child Health
Madras Medical College
Chennai, Tamil Nadu, India

Prophylaxis for Exposure to Diphtheria

Vairam Muthu MD DCH
Assistant Professor
Department of Pediatrics
KAP Viswanathan Government Medical College
Tiruchirapalli, Tamil Nadu, India

How to avoid Catastrophe during CT/MRI?

R Elilarasu MD FPICU
Senior Assistant Professor
Pediatric Intensive Care Department
Institute of Child Health
Madras Medical College
Chennai, Tamil Nadu, India

Hand Washing

Ramesh Babu MD DCH
Associate Professor of Pediatrics
Department of Pediatrics
Government Dharmapuri Medical College
Dharmapuri, Tamil Nadu, India

Clinical Aids and Drug Dosages

Baljit Cheema MBBS, MRCPCH BSc DTM&H
Clinical Lead, Specialized Pediatric Retrieval Including Neonatal Transfer Team
Pediatric Emergency Specialist
Emergency Medical Services
Western Cape Government Health
Senior Lecturer
Division of Emergency Medicine
University of Cape Town
Cape Town, South Africa

Pediatric Emergency Medicine Case Record and Decision-making Steps

J Deepa MD (Pediatrics)
Assistant Surgeon
District Headquarter Hospital
Cuddalore, Tamil Nadu, India

Poisoning

S Sakthi Vel MS
Postgraduate
Department of Surgery
Sri Ramachandra Medical College and Research Institute
Chennai, Tamil Nadu, India

Cover Design and PREM Logo

Foreword

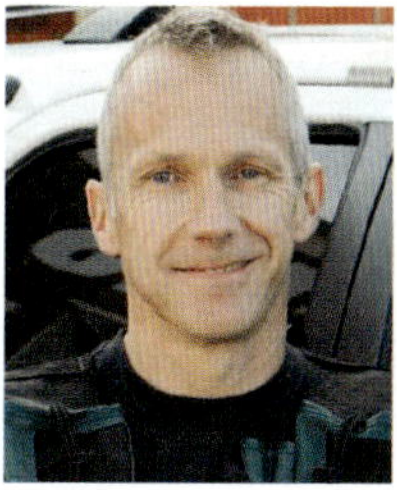

India has the largest child population in the world, and with this comes one of the world's greatest burdens of pediatric disease. Indeed, this burden may seem overwhelming. India has made remarkable progress in reducing its rates of under-5 and neonatal mortality; yet more will be need to be done in order to achieve the targets set by the UN Sustainable Development Goals. The main drivers of child morbidity and mortality in this setting—trauma, pneumonia, diarrhea are presentations which are addressed by emergency care. In fact, it is estimated that emergency care can save around half of the deaths in lower resourced settings each year, a great many of whom are children.

This is therefore the ideal moment for an update of the Pediatric Emergency Medicine Course (PEMC). It is essential that the pediatric disease burden is tackled by experienced, well-trained emergency health workers. And while there is no substitute for experience, this well-constructed volume provides a high standard of pediatric emergency training. The overwhelming majority of existing pediatric emergency training manuals focus on high-income settings and are premised on the availability of resources that simply do not exist in many parts of the world. It gives me great pleasure, therefore, to endorse the PEMC in this new iteration. This course exactly fills that gap with recommendations and guidance that are appropriate to not only the Indian context, but also much more widely—the challenges faced by those working with limited resources are the same in much of the world.

I look forward to seeing the progress that will be made with the help of the PEMC over the coming years. Congratulations to the editors and authors on a very valuable product!

Lee Wallis Close MBChB MD Dip IMC RCS Edin Dip Sport Med FRCS Edin FRCP Edin FRCEM FCEM(SA) FEMSSA FIFEM
President, International Federation for Emergency Medicine
Immediate Past President, African Federation for Emergency Medicine
Head of Emergency Medicine, Western Cape Government
Professor and Head of Emergency Medicine
Stellenbosch University, Stellenbosch
Professor and Head of Emergency Medicine
University of Cape Town, Cape Town, South Africa

Preface

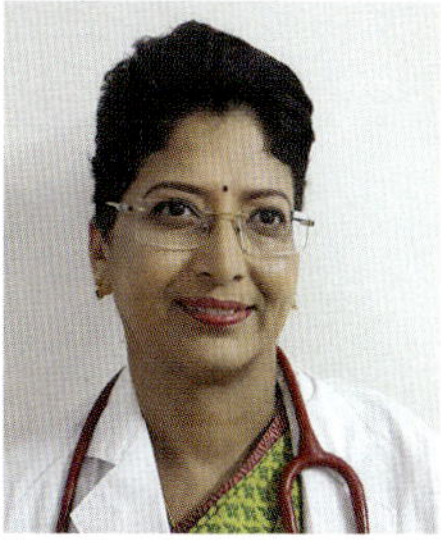

The entrance of hospitals in India, is often manned by novice doctors fresh out of medical school who are inexperienced in providing pediatric emergency care. Indeed, a white paper published by the Indian Academy of Pediatrics in 2015, reported that the concept of pediatric emergency medicine (PEM) is virtually nonexistent in India. With the failure of the Medical Council of India to include, PEM in its under-graduate curriculum, young doctors are woefully unprepared when they encounter a critically ill or injured child.

Based on the experience gained from training house officers and under-graduates in the field of PEM, over the past 2 decades, this pocket manual shows how to save life in simple systematic steps in the absence of trained emergency physicians.

Advanced interventions, such as pericardiocentesis or thoracocentesis, thoracotomy, etc. are beyond the scope of the manual.

An innovative case record has been devised which aids in assessment, intervention and documentation during resuscitation. The pediatric assessment triangle has been simplified to assist decision making. A color atlas, shows how to mask ventilate, introduce a laryngeal mask airway (LMA) or secure intraosseous access. In addition, information has been added about common drugs used in the out patient department, prophylaxis following exposure, procedures, approach to fever and how to prepare one-self when shifting a child for radiology.

Indumathy Santhanam MD DCH
Professor of Pediatrics
Head, Department of Pediatric
Emergency Medicine
Institute of Child Health
Madras Medical College
Chennai, Tamil Nadu, India

Acknowledgments

Success in resuscitation is hugely dependent on team effort. The Pocket Pediatric Emergency Medicine Course (PEMC) for Interns is no exception.

I thank, Dr Murali, Dr Balaji, Dr Ramesh Babu and Dr Chandan Kumar who share a passion for this specialty and who have contributed important sections for the manual. I also thank, Dr Akila Sivakumar, Dr Sharada Sathish, Dr Shanthi and Dr Jayanthi, the PEMC editorial team who toiled tirelessly to edit and correct the proofs.

I am deeply grateful for to Dr Gundas Srinivasan, who made several trips to New Delhi to coordinate with the publishing team on the presentation of this book. In the process, he helped design the decision-making triangle, an important resource developed for this manual.

I thank, Dr Sakthivel for designing the beautiful cover page for this manual. Without his instantaneous and amazing creativity, we would not have been able to complete this project on time.

I also thank, Dr Sakthi Vel, for designing the PREM logo. The lotus is an Egyptian symbol of resurrection. The Celtic symbol indicates the indestructible bond between mother and child. The overall choice of colors is from the Indian flag, with special emphasis on saffron, a color that denotes the sacrifice needed to save young lives.

My special thanks to Dr Baljit Cheema, who passionately believes that this resource could help a larger group of physicians in Africa. Her insights have helped construct a simple case record that would aid in making therapeutic decisions.

Words cannot express how grateful I am to all the parents who entrusted their most precious possession to our care and who stood with us as we resuscitated, taught and documented the treatment given to children. I thank all the parents for consenting to use the photographs for educational purposes.

I am grateful to my parents, my husband Dr Ramesh Dorairajan, my daughter Dr Varshini Ramesh, sister Subhashini and brother JP for their constant encouragement and support.

I would also like to thank, Mr Jitendar P Vij (Group Chairman), Ms Chetna Malhotra Vohra (Associate Director—Content Strategy), Ms Payal Bharti and Mr Jayanandan for their tireless efforts in making this dream come true.

Contents

1

CHAPTER

Recognition of Critical Illness

Chapter Outline

Recognition of hypoxia, shock, cardiac dysfunction and non-convulsive status epilepticus in the child brought to the OPD

TRIAGE: SERIOUSLY ILL OR NOT?

Triage is the method of recognizing whether a child brought to the OPD, is very sick or not. Snake envenomation, toxin ingestion, accidents, drowning, etc. are easily recognized as "bad history" and rapidly shifted into the emergency department (ED).

- *How do we recognize hypoxia and shock in children brought with "routine symptoms" such as fever, diarrhea vomiting or any focus of infection?*
- *An acute fall in mental status is one of the earliest symptoms of hypoxia and shock.*

APPEARANCE

The severity of level of consciousness (LOC) or "appearance" is rapidly evaluated using the AVPU scale.

Alert (A)

"Alert", is based on mother's perception that her child is "as usual". It is based on her history that he is inter-acting normally, is playfulness or is consolable.

Responsive to Voice (V)

- *Recognition of drop in mental status from alert to "responsive to voice" is not easy. Take mom's help to find out whether her child is ok or not?*
- *History of inconsolable cry, lethargy, "more sleepy than usual" or "not as usual" in a child presenting with acute diarrhea, fever or breathlessness suggests hypoxia or shock.*

- Even if the child looks "alert", remember, mom knows best! If she feels the child is not alright, she is probably right!
- Perform the rapid cardiopulmonary cerebral assessment.

Responsive to Pain (P)

- Sudden flexor or extensor stiffening associated with an upward gaze or hypotonia in a neurologically normal child with breathlessness, fever or diarrhea may be secondary to respiratory failure or shock.

> - *Posturing secondary to hypoxia and hypoperfusion is often mistaken as status epilepticus.*

- Anti-seizure medications, could have lethal effects when posturing occurs secondary to severe hypoxia or/and shock.
- In older children with fever, diarrhea or breathlessness, lethargy, inability to sit, stand or walk, agitation, fighting the oxygen mask, abusive behavior or combativeness suggest cerebral hypoperfusion or shock.

Unresponsiveness (U)

> - *The commonest cause of sudden unresponsiveness in the absence of precipitating events in a previously normal child or a child with seizure disorder is suggestive of non-convulsive status epilepticus.*

BREATHLESSNESS

The commonest causes of respiratory distress are bronchiolitis, pneumonia and asthma. However, severe insults due to drowning, prolonged status epilepticus, severe sepsis, scorpion venom can also cause respiratory distress. These insults can directly affect the heart and the vessels (Figure 1).

Hypoxia, cytokine storm, venom, etc. can cause vasodilation and capillary leak in both the systemic and pulmonary circulation.

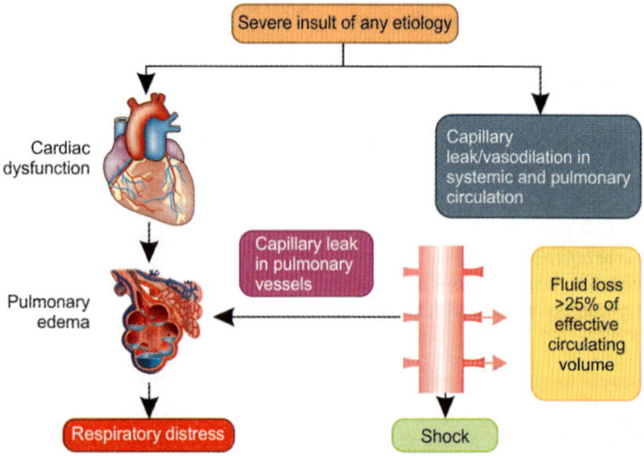

Figure 1: Shocked children often present with respiratory distress.

When, more than 25% of effective circulatory volume is lost, shock occurs. At the same time, the capillary leak in the pulmonary circulation causes noncardiogenic pulmonary edema. The same insults also directly affect the heart! Myocardial dysfunction also causes cardiogenic pulmonary edema.

TRIAGE QUESTIONS

1. Does your child with fever, diarrhea, cough, cold, etc. have drop in mental status? If yes, consider shock.
2. Does your child, with fever or diarrhea, etc. also have breathlessness?

If yes, confirm whether the breathlessness is present since early infancy (? congestive heart failure) or whether it is episodic in nature? (? Asthma or recurrent aspiration)

If fall in mental status or breathlessness is confirmed, perform the following assessment.

RAPID CARDIOPULMONARY ASSESSMENT

1. A stepwise, systematic method known as the "Rapid Cardiopulmonary Cerebral Assessment" is used to find out whether a child is seriously ill or not.
2. The clinical findings are then incorporated into the pediatric assessment triangle (PAT) (Figure 2).
3. As assessment is being made, life-saving interventions are also implemented without loss of time.

AIRWAY

The airway is the passage that connects the oropharynx to the glottis. This narrow tube is kept open by the inherent tone of the surrounding palatopharyngeal muscles and the tongue. Entry of liquid or solid into this passage, is prevented by "cough" a powerful airway protective reflex. Deglutition reflex is the other reflex that prevents liquid from entering the air passage.

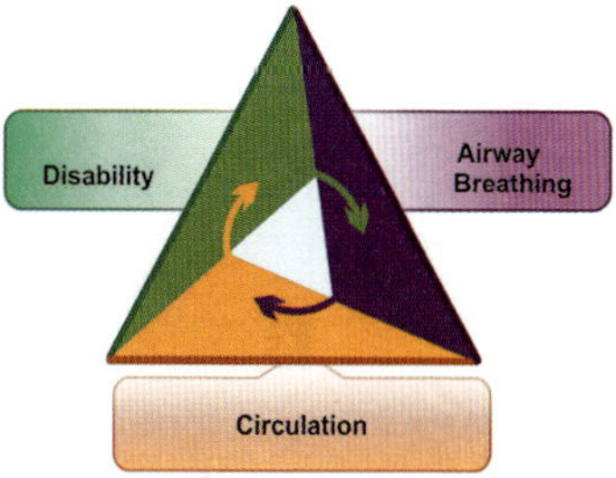

Figure 2: Pediatric assessment triangle.

Maintainable or Stable Airway

- Crying, talking or coughing.

Obstructed Airway: Stridor

- Stridor in an alert child implies the presence of a structural obstruction to the air passage such as glottic edema, foreign body, laryngomalacia, laryngeal web, hemangioma, angioedema, etc.

Unmaintainable Airway

- When a child becomes unresponsive or convulsing the inherent tone of the palate-pharyngeal muscles are lost resulting in collapse and falling back of the tongue (Figures 3A and B). Loss of airway protective reflexes, such as cough and deglutition result in pooling of secretions.

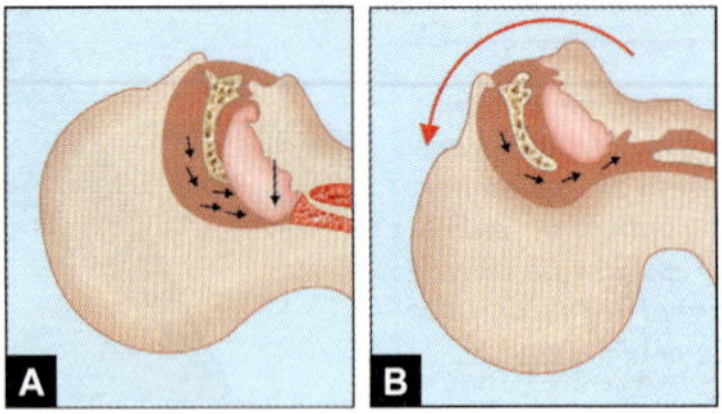

Figures 3A and B: (A) Commonest cause of airway obstruction: Falling back of tongue in unresponsive victim; (B) The head tilt chin lift maneuver aids in relieving the obstruction caused by the tongue.

Obstruction to the airway (tongue or secretions) aggravates hypoxia.

Physiological Status

- Airway is classified as maintainable (crying, talking) obstructed (stridor) or not maintainable.

Airway Management

- If crying or stridor is noted, the child may be assessed and managed on the mother's lap.

Avoid separating the mother and child, if the airway is maintainable or obstructed (crying or have stridor)

If the child is unresponsive with or without posturing or fits, he should be placed on the resuscitation trolley.

1. Open the airway using the head tilt chin lift maneuver (Figure 4).

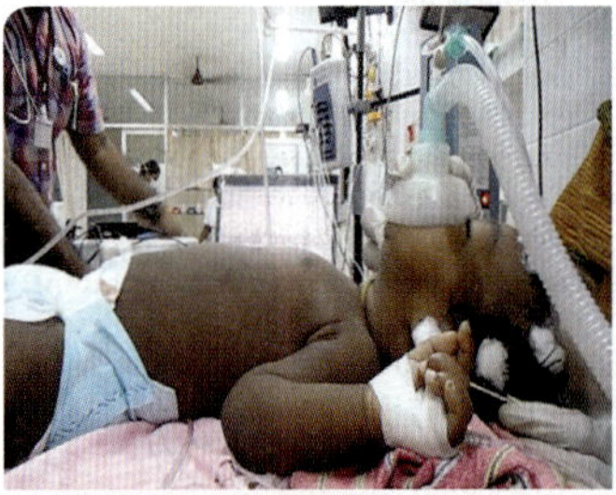

Figure 4: This unresponsive child is unable to sit or stand since he has lost his tone and posture. It is presumed, that the internal tone of the palate-pharyngeal muscles and tongue is also lost resulting in falling back of the tongue (obstruction of the air-passage). In addition, he has also lost the ability to cough, cry or swallow (airway protective reflexes).

2. Suction oropharyngeal secretions, if noted.
3. Insert an age appropriate nasogastric tube and decompress stomach (to avoid risk of aspiration).

BREATHING

1. Breathing is assessed by counting respiratory rate for 6 seconds and multiplying by 10 (Figure 5).

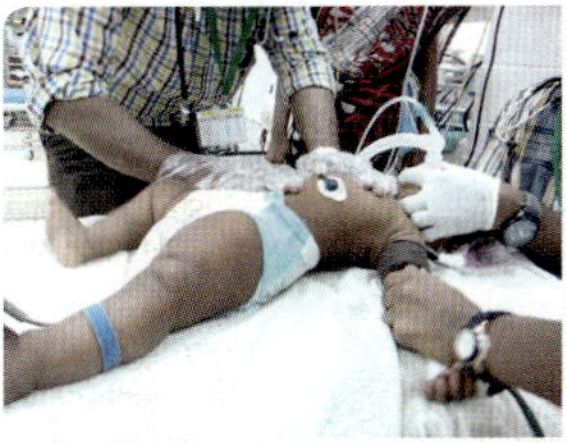

Figure 5: Both hands are placed, one on the thorax and the other on the abdomen, to assess whether thoracic respiration or abdominal respiration.

2. If not breathing or respiratory rate is in the lower range for normal in the unresponsive child, initiate bag valve mask ventilation. The 2nd responder will continue the assessment.
3. If the child is tachypneic, the assessment is continued; While counting respiratory rate, the work of breathing must be concurrently noted. Is the child having retractions, grunt, abdominothoracic or thoracic respiration? (grunt and abdominal respiration are suggestive of impending respiratory failure).
4. Auscultate the infra-axillary region for air-entry and added sounds (all three lobes are represented in this area).
5. Color is evaluated by comparing the palm of the physician with that of the child's sole (Figure 6). Pallor, dusky hue, ashen, mottling is documented as abnormal.

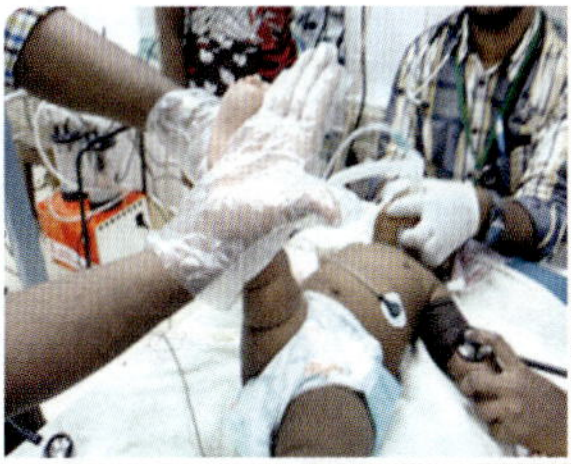

Figure 6: Comparing the color of physician's palm with the color of the sole of the child.

Physiological Status

Breathing is classified as:

a. Normal
b. Effortless tachypnea
c. Respiratory distress
d. Impending respiratory failure
e. Apnea

Management of Breathing

1. Apnea: Bag valve mask ventilation is initiated.
2. Effortless tachypnea: Oxygen is provided using a nonrebreathing mask.
3. Respiratory distress or impending respiratory failure: Oxygen is provided using a flow inflating ventilation device (Jackson-Rees circuit).

   If the child is breathing spontaneously, the assessment is continued.

CIRCULATION

Heart rate is assessed for 6 seconds and multiplied by 10 (Figure 7).

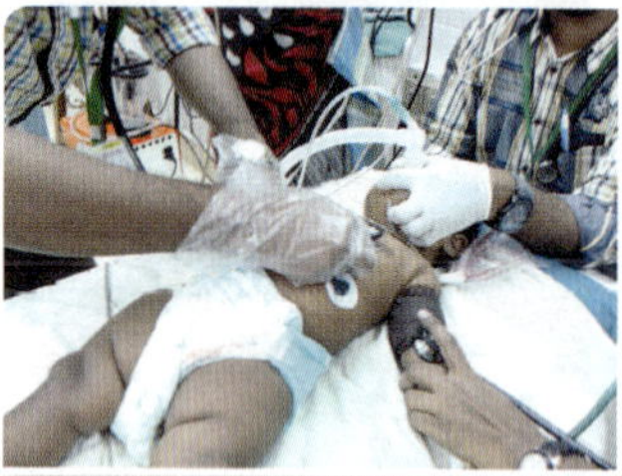

Figure 7: Assessment of both heart rate and quality of heart sounds.

If heart sounds are difficult to hear, or heart rate is in the lower range of normal in the unresponsive child with apnea, chest compressions are initiated in the ratio of 15: 2 (Figure 8).

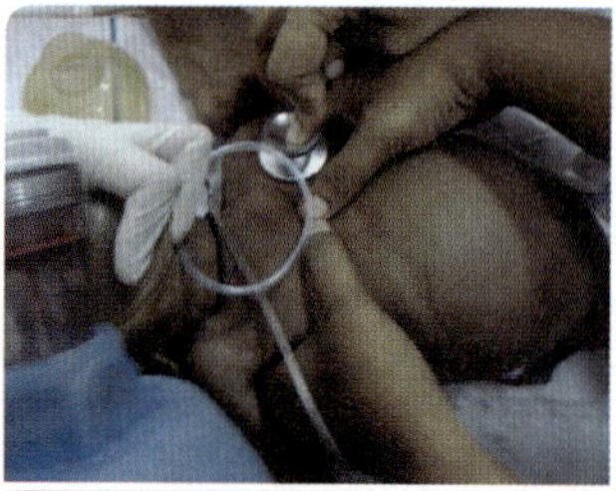

Figure 8: Initiating chest compression in a young infant.

(The 1st responder should have already initiated bag valve mask ventilation). A 3rd responder continues with the assessment.

Heart sounds should also be assessed for gallop or muffling (ominous signs). If tachycardic, the peripheral perfusion is evaluated.

Tachycardia is the earliest sign of hypoxia or shock.

Since this sign can be precipitated by anxiety or stranger distress, children with patent airway and spontaneous breathing must be evaluated in their mom's lap with minimal disturbance.

1. Compare core and peripheral temperature by placing the dorsum of one hand on the abdomen and sliding the other hand over the thigh, knee and the ankle (Figure 9).

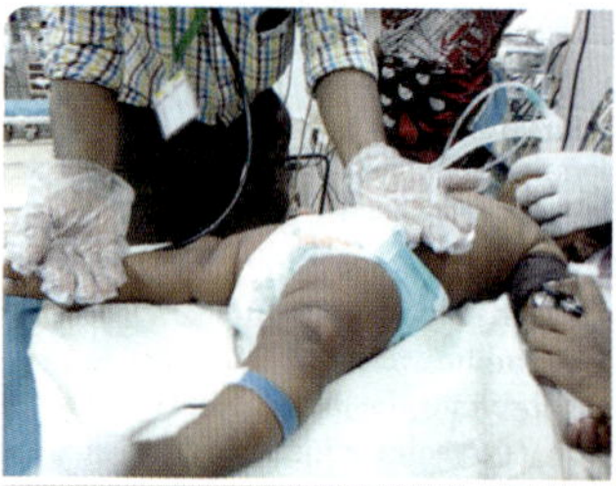

Figure 9: Comparison of core-peripheral temperature.

Table 1: Comparison of femoral and dorsalis pedis.

Femorals	Dorsalis pedis	Pulse pressure	Inference
+++	++	30-40 mm Hg	Normal
+++	+++	> 40 mm Hg	Bounding (vasodilation)
+++	+	< 40	Shock
++	0	Low SBP	Hypotension

Legends:
+++: Easy to feel femorals, ++: Difficult to feel femoral
++: Easy to feel dorsalis pedis, +++: dorsalis pedis as well felt as femoral pulse
+: Just felt dorsalis pedis, 0: not felt dorsalis,
SBP: Systolic Blood Pressure

2. Compare the strength of the femoral (central pulses) with the strength of the dorsalis pedis (peripheral pulse) (Figure 10 and Table 1).

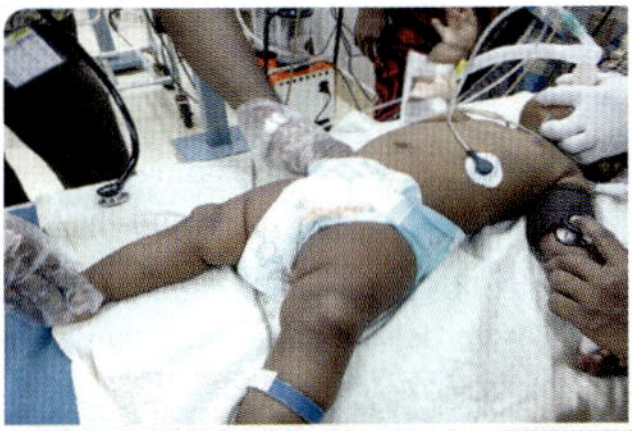

Figure 10: Comparison of femoral pulse with dorsalis pedis.

3. The capillary refill time is assessed by lifting the extremity slightly above the level of the heart and applying enough pressure to blanch the skin (Figure 11). Normal CRT is 2 seconds or less. A prolonged CRT may be seen in shock, rising fever or a cold ambient temperature and is also influenced by lighting, site and age.

4. Color is assessed by comparing the palm of the physician with the color of the child's sole.
5. Assess BP using age appropriate cuffs.

Cuff sizes that are larger than 75% of length between olecranon and elbow can result in false identification of lower BP for age. Cuffs that are smaller, can fail to pick up hypotension.

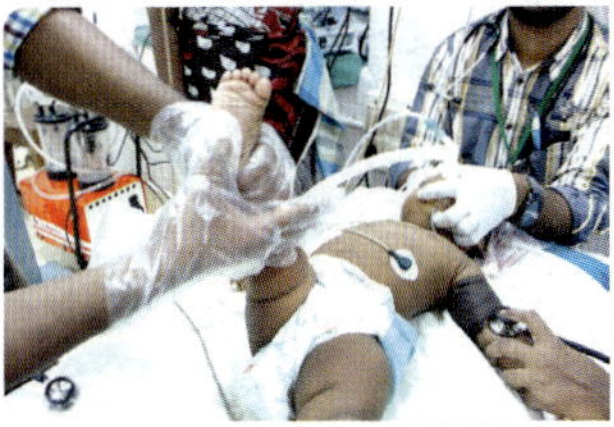

Figure 11: Blanching skin to assess for capillary refill time. It is essential to elevate limb above the level of the heart.

Table 2: Hypotensive (5th percentile) range of blood pressure for age

Term newborn (0–28 day)	SBP < 60 mm Hg
For infant < 12 months	< 70 mm Hg
1–10 years	SBP 70 + (2 × age)
> 10 years	SBP < 90 mm Hg

6. In early shock, children compensate by pushing up their BP (similar to tachycardia). As shock worsens, systolic pressures fall to the normal range. In children who are responsive to pain or unresponsive, BP that is within the lower normal range for age is dangerous (Table 2).

When systolic BP falls to the 5th percentile of systolic pressure as shown in the Table 2, there is a tremendous risk of rapidly progressing to cardiac arrest.

When the diastolic pressure is less than 50% of systolic pressure it is suggestive of vasodilatory shock.

Mean arterial pressure (MAP) is calculated as the sum of the diastolic pressure and one-third pulse pressure.

Wide pulse pressure in association with altered mental status, abnormal respiratory rates, abnormal work of breathing, tachycardia, warm, pink peripheries, bounding pulses and rapid CRT is diagnostic of warm shock.

Conventionally, documentation of systolic pressure is given importance. Early warm shock could be missed, if diastolic pressure and MAP are not noted.

Liver Span

Often, in children with shock, the heart is failing. Pulmonary congestion secondary to cardiac dysfunction manifests as respiratory distress (common symptom of serious illness). Coexisting hepatomegaly, is useful in finding out whether respiratory distress is due to a primary respiratory cause or cardiac dysfunction. The upper border of liver is identified by percussion (Figure 12A) and the lower border by palpation (Figure 12B) and the total span is marked (Figure 12C) and measured in the evaluation of serious illness (Figure 12D).

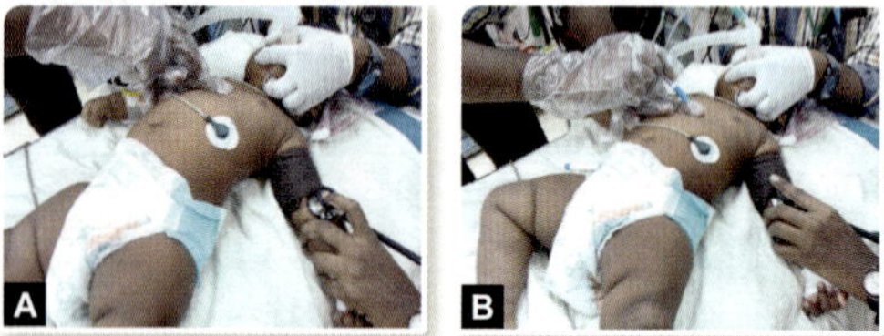

Figures 12A and B:

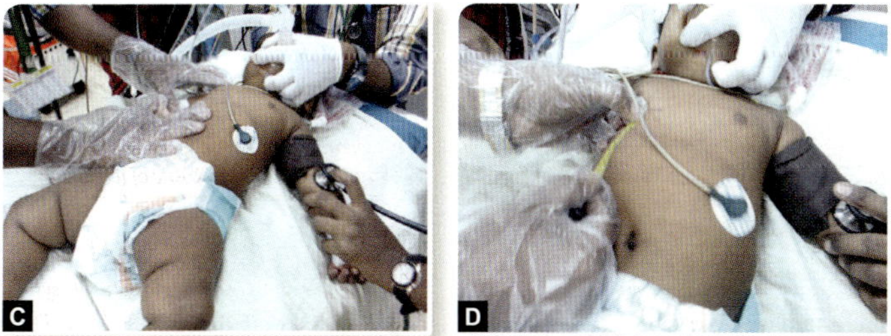

Figures 12A to D: How do we measure liver span. (A) Percuss for upper border for liver; (B) Mark upper border of liver dullness; (C) Palpate for lower border of liver from below upwards. The hand should be placed parallel to the right costal margin. Mark the lower border of liver; (D) Measure the distance between the 2 lines.

Respiratory distress + hepatomegaly=? Cardiac dysfunction with pulmonary edema

Physiological Status

Circulation is classified as:

- Heart rate: Normal/tachycardia/relative bradycardia/bradycardia,
- Perfusion: Normal/shock
- Hepatomegaly: Yes/No
- BP: Normal/ high/low
- MAP: Normal/low.

Management of Circulation

1. If bradycardic, chest compressions are initiated. Refer to BLS section
2. If tachycardic shock
   a. Secure IV/IO
   b. Type of fluid: Administer isotonic nonglucose containing fluids such as normal saline (NS) or Ringer's lactate (RL)
   c. Volume: 20 ml/kg
   d. Break 20 ml/kg to smaller aliquots of 5–10 ml/kg, if shock is associated with respiratory distress.
   Mark the calculated volume on the bottle containing the fluid to avoid excess fluid administration.
   e. Rate: over 20 minutes by gravity (the stop. The calculated dose of fluids runs by gravity cock in the IV tubing should be fully open).
   If tachycardic and hypotensive for age use pull push technique to rapidly infuse fluids (Figures 13A to C).

DISABILITY

An acute onset of altered behavior, incoherent speech, agitation or fighting the mask in children with history of fever, diarrhea, etc.

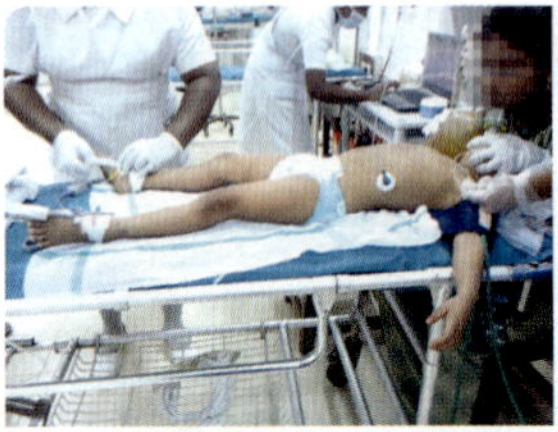

Figure 13A: The 3-way stop cock that is being used to withdraw aliquots of fluids from the bottle and pushed into the patient while bagging is in progress.

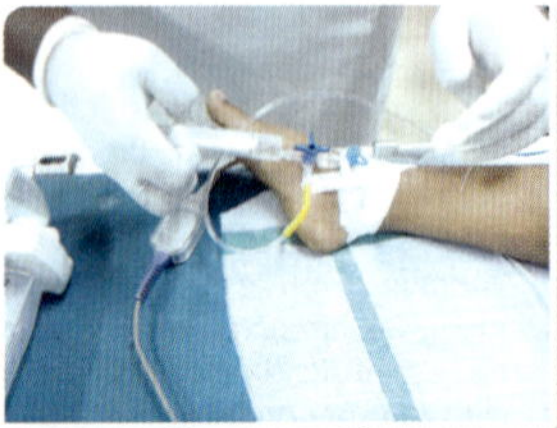

Figure 13C: Pull-push technique is used to rapidly administer NS or RL in the shortest possible time.
Note that the 3 way has been turned to permit NS push into the patient end. The reservoir end has been blocked.

is indicative of severe cerebral hypoxia or cerebral hypoperfusion.

In such children consider deep unconsciousness. Failure to aggressively resuscitate these kids could result in rapid deterioration to cardiac arrest!

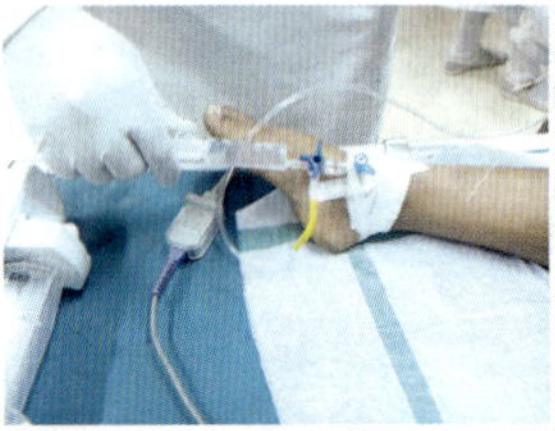

Figure 13B: Note that the 3-way has been turned to permit aspiration of NS from the bottle. The patient end has been blocked.

Unresponsiveness

Loss of consciousness and generalized tonic clonic seizures is a common pediatric emergency (Refer section of Status epilepticus). Conjugate eye deviation, nystagmus or eyelid twitch may indicate subtle seizures or hypoxic ischemic compromise of the brain from shock.

Unequal pupils (Figure 14) may often be noted from increased intracranial pres-

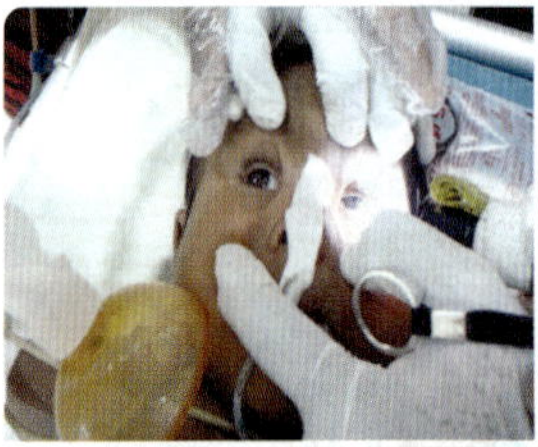

Figure 14: Noting eyes for position and movements while concurrently evaluating pupillary response to light.

sure or nonconvulsive status. Pupils provide important information regarding response to therapy and normalization of abnormal pupillary size, reaction or symmetry indicates resolution of cerebral hypoperfusion and hypoxia.

PHYSIOLOGICAL STATUS

- ALC (due to hypoxia or shock)
- Non-convulsive status epilepticus/Convulsive status epilepticus.
- Raised intra-cranial pressure (ICP)

DO NOT EVER FORGET GLUCOSE (DEFG)

Even as the assessment and life-saving interventions are being provided, capillary glucose levels must be checked and documented in all seriously ill-children.

- If hypoglycemic, rapidly correct with 2 ml/kg of 25% dextrose if Capillary blood glucose is less than 60 mg/dl.

Temperature

Concurrently, temperature is also checked and documented.

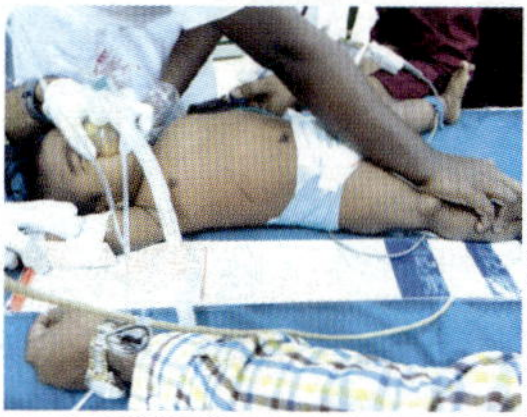

Figure 15: Broselow's tape is being used to measure the approximate weight.

Assess weight using the Broselow's tape (Figure 15)

Measure length, using this tape. The approximate weight for length is marked on this tape.

Exposure

As the child is being assessed, clothes should be removed to pick up other significant clinical findings.

Documentation

- Findings should be documented within 30 seconds.
- The time of assessment must be documented.

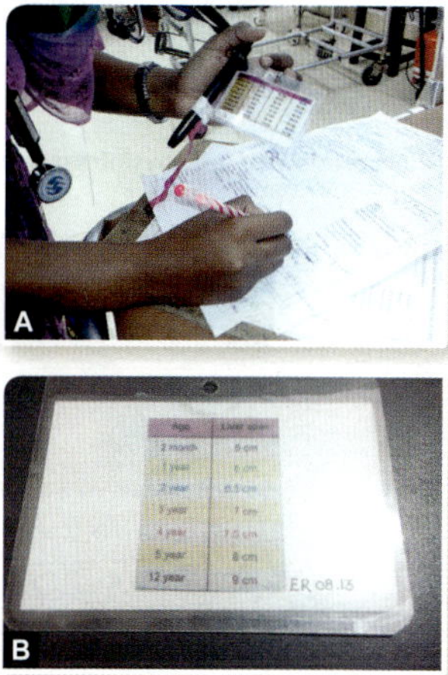

Figures 16A and B:

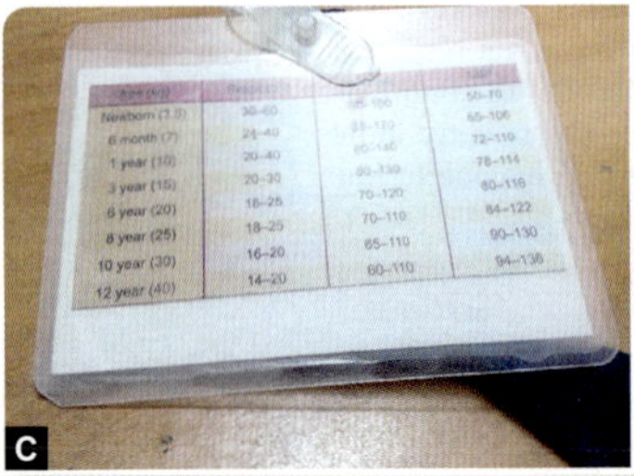

Figures 16A to C: A. Check the vital signs card to interpret the vital signs in relation to the other parts of the pediatric assessment triangle (absolutely low, relatively low or increased); B and C. Card with vital signs and liver span for age.

- Respiratory rates, heart rates, BP and liver span measurements must be counterchecked with a card containing vital signs for age (Figures 16A to C).
- The findings are now inserted into the pediatric assessment triangle to help understand the physiological status. The findings are interpreted based on the other parts of the PAT (Figure 17).

Interpretation of the physiological status using the Pediatric Assessment Triangle

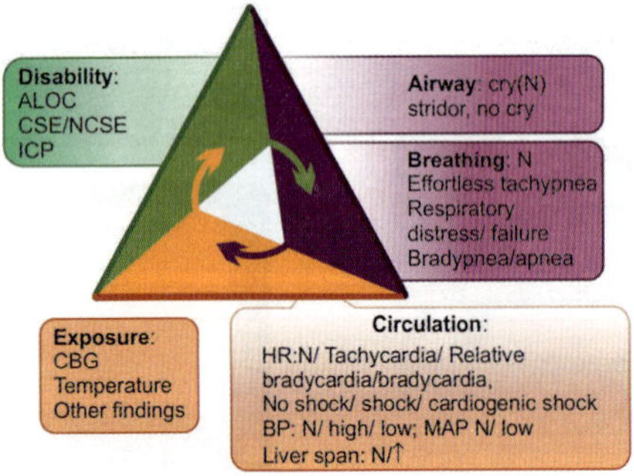

Figure 17: Interpretation of the physiological status using the PAT.

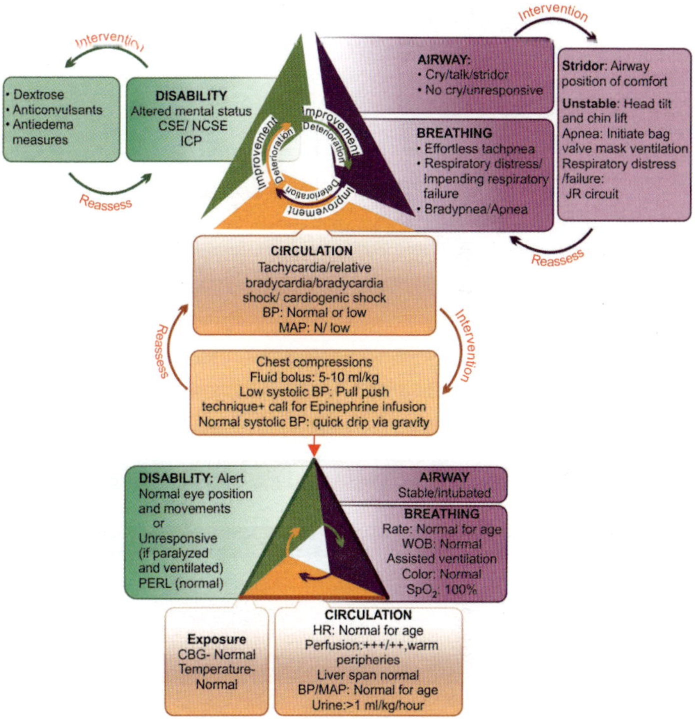

Figure 18: How to perform life saving interventions based on physiological status until therapeutic goals are achieved.

Rapid history				Details
	Yes	No	Duration	
Breathlessness				
Convulsions/Posturing				
Fever				
ALOC				
Scorpion/snakebite				
Toxin/trauma				
Foreign body				Co-morbidities
Jaundice				
AWD/vomiting/GI bleed				
Refusal of feeds				Drugs/Allergies
Abdominal pain/distension				
Bad CRP/bottle feed				

Airway

Initial assessment:				
Stable	Unstable		Obstructed	
Immediate Management:				
O2	NRM	BVM	JR	ETT

Breathing

Initial assessment:			RR/min
Nasal flaring	Grunting	Stridor	Retractions
Thoracic breathing	Abdominal breathing		Air entry R
Crepitations	Wheeze		Air entry L
Colour	O2 sat		
Immediate management – record dose & time			
Nebulised salbutamol/ipratropium		Prednisolone	
Epinephrine	Neb	I.M.	Hydrocortisone

Circulation

Initial assessment:					HR/min
Heart sounds	Normal		Muffled		Gallop
Pulse volume	Femoral	+++	++	+	0
	DP	+++	++	+	0
Skin temperature	Warm	Below thigh	Below knee	Below ankle	
	Cool	Below thigh	Below knee	Below ankle	
CRT ____ seconds	Liver span		BP		
Immediate management – record volume/dose & time commenced					
Fluids	Inotropes:		Other:		

Disability

Initial assessment	Alert		Voice		Pain	Unaresponsive
RIGHT Pupil size ______ mm Reactive Yes/No				LEFT Pupil size _____ mm Reactive Yes/No		
EYE Position	Mid-point	Deviated	Nystagmus	Lid twitch	Dolls Eye Yes/No	EOM
GTCS			Focal seizure			
Immediate management – record drug, dose & time given						
Prior treatment:			Treatment initiated now:			

From the Initial Assessment Decide the Patient's Initial Physiological Status for AB/C/D

<table>
<tr><td>A</td><td colspan="2">Stable</td><td colspan="2">Unstable</td><td colspan="2">Obstructed</td></tr>
<tr><td>B</td><td>Normal</td><td>Effortless tachypnoea</td><td>Respiratory distress</td><td>Respiratory failure</td><td>Relative bradypnoea</td><td>Apnoea</td></tr>
</table>

<table>
<tr><td rowspan="3">C</td><td>HR normal</td><td>Tachycardia</td><td colspan="2">Bradycardia</td><td colspan="2">Relative bradycardia</td></tr>
<tr><td colspan="2">Perfusion:
Cold/slow CRT
Warm/flushed</td><td rowspan="2">BP</td><td>Systolic</td><td>Diastolic</td><td>Pulse pressure:</td></tr>
<tr><td>Shock with normal liver span</td><td>Shock INCREASED liver span</td><td>Normal
Low
High</td><td>Normal
Low
High</td><td>Normal

Wide</td></tr>
</table>

D	Normal	ALOC	GTC Seizure	Focal Seizure	CSE	NCSE	Raised ICP

See Chart 1: Match AB/C/D to correct triangle => manage as per guidance then reassess

Time									
Symptoms									
Airway									
RR									
Grunt									
Stridor									
Retractions									
Abdominal/Thoracic									
Air entry									
Added sounds									
Color									

SaO_2										
HR										
Central/Distal pulse										
Core-peripheral temperature gap										
CRT										
Liver span										
BP										
AVPU										
Pupils										
Eye position/nystagmus/lid twitch										
DEM/EOM										
Tone/posture										
Seizure										
Urine output										
Physiological status	Airway									
	Breathing									
	Circulation									
	Disability									
Interventions	A&B									
	C									
	D									

Normal triangle

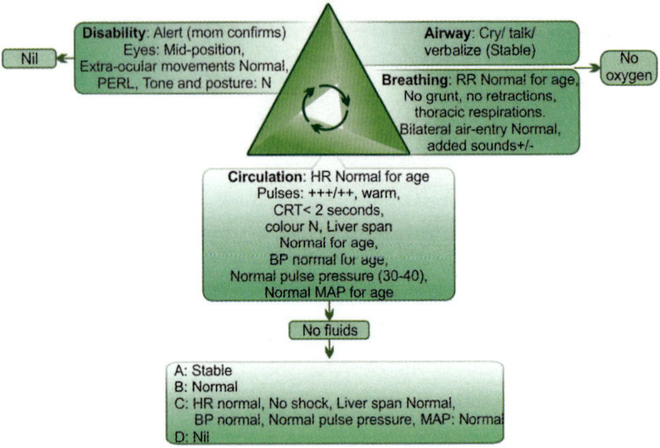

Compensated shock triangle

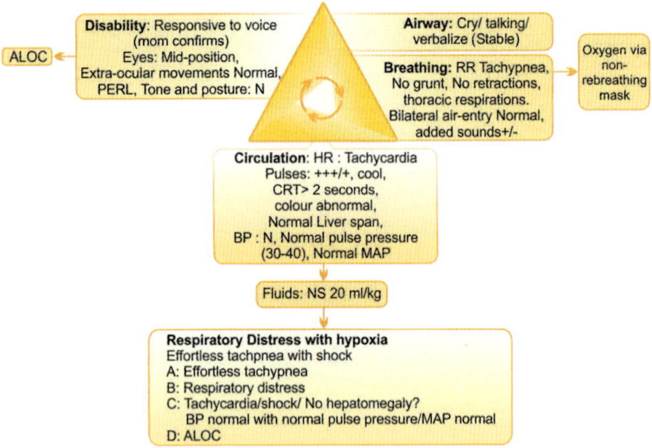

Respiratory distress with some hypoxia triangle

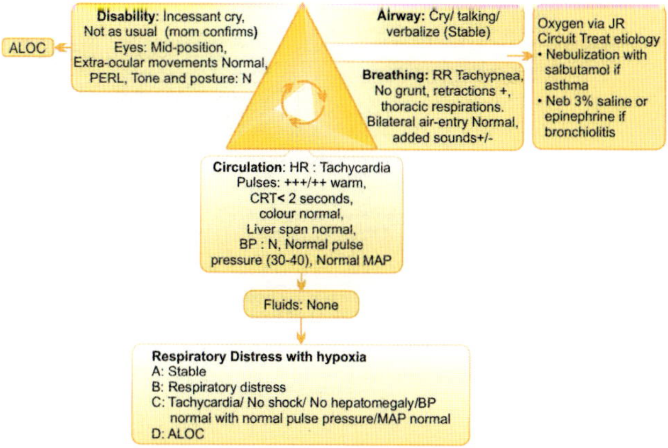

Congesive cardiac failure triangle

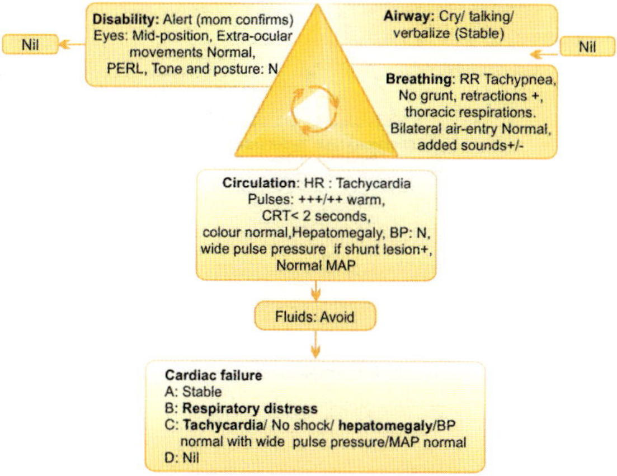

Respiratory distress with normotensive vasodilatory shock triangle

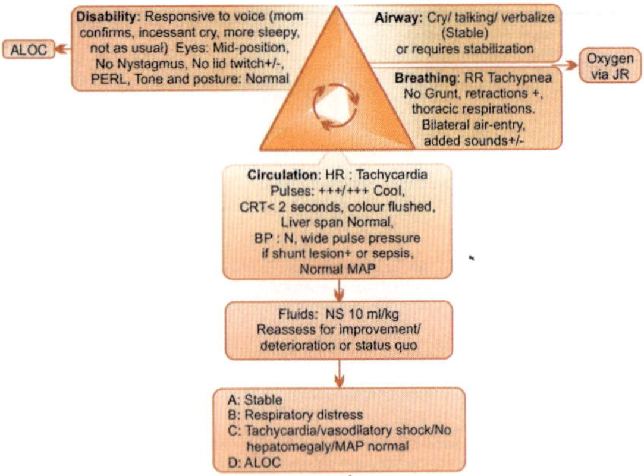

Respiratory failure with normotensive vasodilatory cardiogenic shock triangle

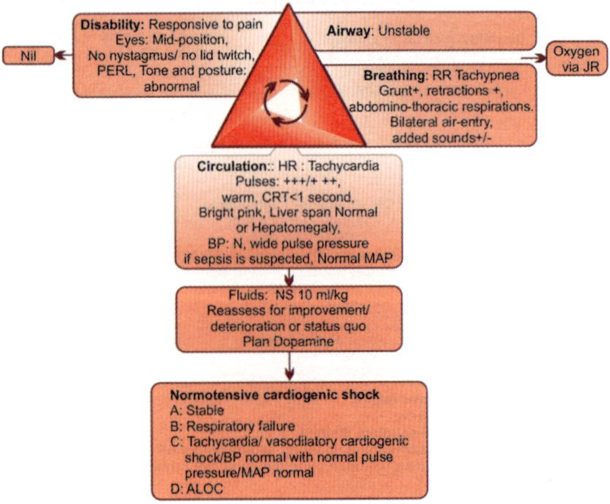

Respiratory arrest with hypotensive cardiogenic shock triangle

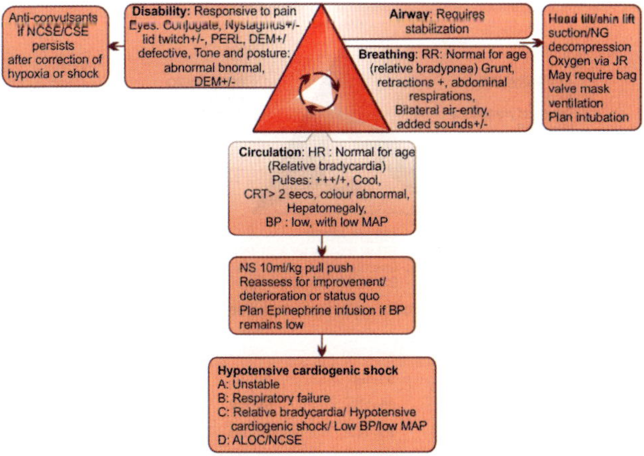

Imminent arrest triangle

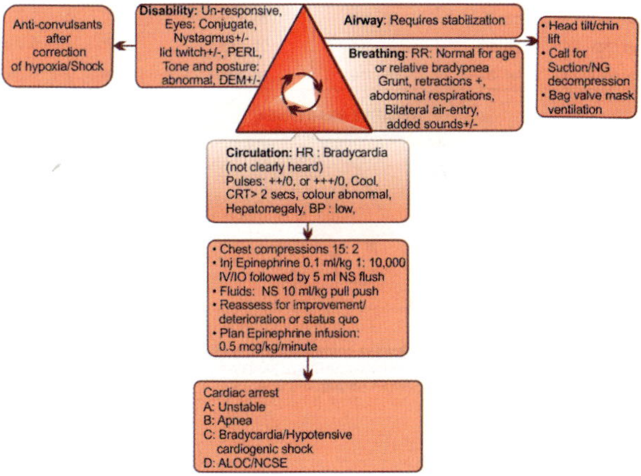

Protocol 1.1: PEMC approach: Recognition of relative bradypnea and relative bradycardia

NORMAL

APPEARANCE
Alert,
Tone and posture: N
Eyes: MP
EOM: N/PERL

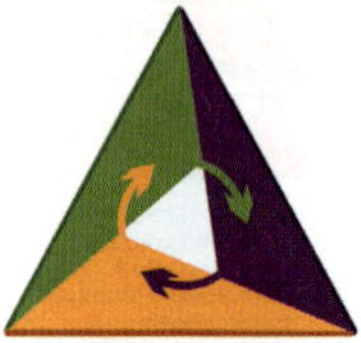

BREATHING
RR: N (for age)
WOB: N
Color: N

CIRCULATION
HR: N (normal for age), Perfusion: N
Liver span: N
BP: N, PP: 30–40 mm Hg

NORMAL VITAL SIGNS FOR AGE

Age (kg)	Respiration	Heart rate	SBP
Newborn (3.5)	30–60	90–180	50–70
6 month (7)	24–40	85–170	65–106
1 year (10)	20–40	80–140	72–110
3 year (15)	20–30	80–130	78–114
6 year (20)	18–25	70–120	80–116
8 year (25)	18–25	70–110	84–122
10 year (30)	16–20	65–110	90–130
12 year (40)	14–20	60–110	94–136

Age	Liver span
2 month	5 cm
1 year	6 cm
2 year	6.5 cm
3 year	7 cm
4 year	7.5 cm
5 year	8 cm
12 year	9 cm

RELATIVE BRADYPNEA
IMMINENT ARREST

APPEARANCE
Pain responsive or
unresponsive
Posturing/floppy
Eye: Deviated laterally/upward/
Nystagmus: +/-, Lid twitch: +/-,
PERL: Sluggish

BREATHING
RR: Normal for age
WOB: ↓
Initiate bag-valve-mask ventilation

CIRCULATION
Relative bradycardia (HR: N for age)
Perfusion: ++/0, cyanosis/cool peripheries, CRT > 2 sec
hepatomegaly, BP: Low
Initiate chest compressions, call for epinephrine

Protocol 1.2: PEMC approach: Recognition of severity of illness on arrival to the ED

NORMAL

APPEARANCE
Alert
Tone : N
Posture : N
Eyes : MP
EOM : N

BREATHING
RR : N
WOB : N
Breath sounds : N

CIRCULATION
Heart rate: N
Perfusion: CRT < 2 sec
Warm peripheries: Pink, +++/++
Liver span: N
BP: N, PP: 30–40 mm Hg

[illegible]

APPEARANCE
Alert
Tone : N
Posture : N
Eyes : MP
EOM : N

OTHERS
Temperature:
< 36.5°C or > 38°C
Focus of infection

BREATHING
RR: > 2 SD for age
WOB : N
Breath sounds : N

CIRCULATION
HR: > 2 SD for age,
Perfusion: CRT < 2 sec
Warm peripheries: Pink, +++/++
Liver span: N
BP: N, PP: 30–40 mm Hg

RESPIRATORY DISTRESS

Alert
Eyes: MP
EOM: N
Tone/
posture: N

RR: ↑
WOB: ↑

HR: ↑/N
Perfusion: N
Liver span: N
BP: N, PP: 30–40 mm Hg

CARDIAC FAILURE

Alert
Eyes: MP
EOM: N
Tone and
posture: N

RR: ↑
WOB: ↑
Crepts: +/-

HR: ↑
Perfusion: N
Liver span: ↑
BP: N PP: 30–40 mm Hg

COMPENSATED SHOCK

V/P/U
Eyes: MP
EOM: N
Tone and
posture: N

RR: ↑
WOB: N/↑

HR: ↑
Perfusion: ↓
Liver span: N
BP: N/↑
BP: N, PP: 30–40 mm Hg

RESPIRATORY FAILURE

Impaired alert
Inconsolable
Pain responsive: Abn
Eye deviation
Nystagmus: +/-
Lid twitch: +/-

RR: ↑/↓
WOB: ↑/↓

HR: ↑/↓
Perfusion: Abn
Liver span: N

CARDIOGENIC SHOCK

Impaired alert
Inconsolable cry
Pain responsive
Tone/posture: Abn
Deviation: +/-
Nystagmus: +/-
Lid twitch: +/-

RR: ↑/↓
WOB: ↑/↓
Crepts: +

HR: ↑/↓
Perfusion: D
Liver span: N/↑

DECOMPENSATED SHOCK

Impaired alert
Inconsolable cry
Pain responsive
Tone/posture: Abn
Eye deviation: +/-
Nystagmus: +/-
Lid twitch: +/-
GTCS: +/-

Airway:
Unstable
RR: ↑/↓
WOB: ↑/↓

HR: ↑/↓
Perfusion: ↓
BP: ↓
Liver span: N/↑

IMMINENT ARREST

Unresponsive
Posturing/GTC: +/-
Eye deviation: +/-
Nystagmus: +/-
Lid twitch: +/-

Unstable
RR: ↓
WOB: ↓

HR: ↓
Perfusion: ↓
BP: ↓
Liver span: N/↑

Age	Liver span
2 month	5 cm
1 year	6 cm
2 year	6.5 cm
3 year	7 cm
4 year	7.5 cm
5 year	8 cm
12 year	9 cm

KEY POINTS

1. Do not ignore the mom's history of altered mental status. Perform the detailed the rapid assessment.
2. The rapid cardiopulmonary cerebral assessment aids in picking up seriously ill children.
3. If in doubt, give oxygen and one bolus and reassess (treat the mother's history).
4. A high index of suspicion is essential to recognize vasodilatory shock in the appropriate settings.

2

CHAPTER

Approach to Critically Ill Child: Not Breathing Spontaneously or Breathing Spontaneously

Chapter Outline

- Not breathing spontaneously:
  - How do I perform bag valve mask ventilation followed by intubation?
  - How do I provide ventilation when I do not know how to intubate in pre-hospital settings?
  - Laryngeal mask airway (LMA)
- Breathing spontaneously:
  - What oxygen delivery device do I use in the critically ill child presenting with breathlessness?

NOT BREATHING SPONTANEOUSLY

BAG VALVE MASK VENTILATION (SELF-INFLATING VENTILATION DEVICE)

Key to successful bag mask ventilation comprises of 4 steps

Introduction

Self-inflating bag valve mask devices are used to initiate respiratory support in apneic children. It is designed to deliver positive pressure breaths when compressed.

Key to successful bag mask ventilation comprises of 4 steps:

Preparation of Patient

a. Open the airway using the head tilt chin lift maneuver
b. Prior to initiating bag vale mask BVM) ventilation, suction the oropharynx using a large bore Yankauer suction catheter. The Yankauer catheter has a wide bore tip that aids in clearing large volume vomitus and food particles rapidly. Avoid stimulation of the posterior pharynx during suctioning by turning the head to one side. This simple maneuver prevents vagal induced bradycardia.
c. Simultaneously, empty stomach contents by rapidly introducing a large bore nasogastric tube, and decompressing the stomach using a suction apparatus.
d. Assess respiratory rate. If apneic, bag valve mask ventilation is initiated.

Selecting the Right-sized Bag (Figure 1)

Most seriously ill children who require respiratory support on arrival into the emergency, have abnormal lung parenchyma.

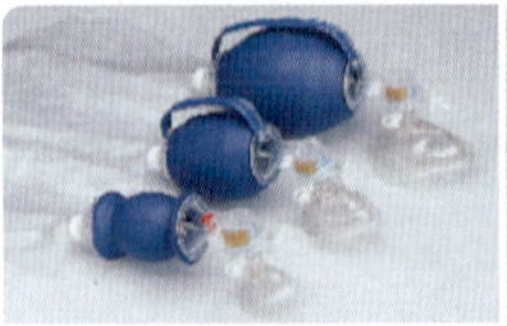

Figure 1: Different sizes of the bag valve masks. Beyond 1 month of age the largest bag is recommended.

Chest compliance is poor and immense effort is often needed to provide effective ventilation and normalize oxygen saturation. The largest bags (1–1.5 liters) are needed to provide effective chest rise. Smaller bags or 'pediatric bags,' i.e. 450 to 750 mL are not sufficient for providing BVM ventilation of critically ill children on arrival into the emergency department (ED).

The largest sized bags should be used in any child beyond the newborn period (Figure 2). 'Regardless of the size of the bag, caution should be taken to use the force and tidal volume to make the chest just visibly rise.'

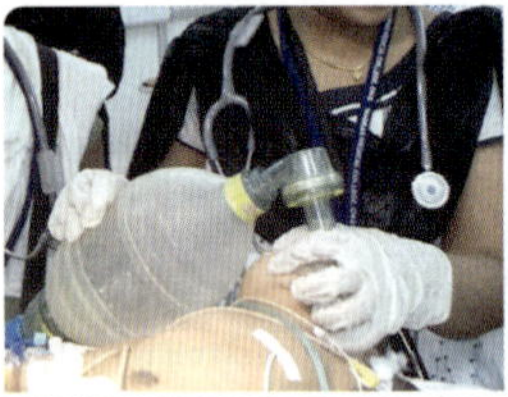

Figure 2: Note that the largest (adult sized bag) is being used to ventilate this infant.

The pop off valve prevents application of pressures greater than 40 cm of water pressure. This precaution is taken to avoid barotrauma in the neonate. In the child beyond the first month of life, higher pressures are needed as mentioned earlier to ventilate bad lungs.

Selecting the Right-sized Mask (Figure 3)

A mask that extends from bridge of nose to chin must be selected. The correct fitting mask is crucial to provide an airtight seal.

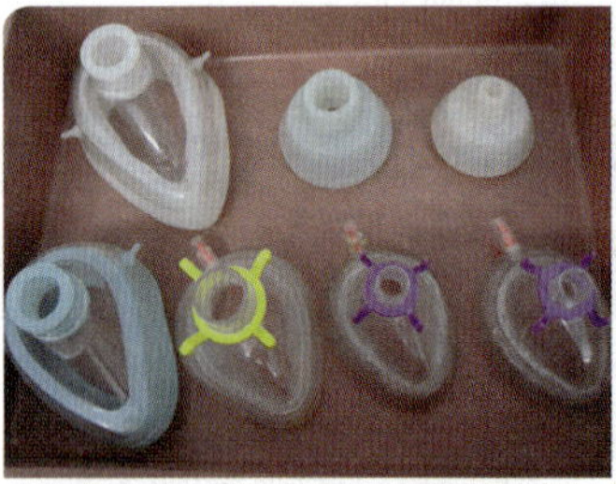

Figure 3: Choosing the right mask is crucial for successful mask ventilation.

The Right Technique

Effective BVM technique may look apparently easy. However, several potentially difficult steps are needed to provide adequate ventilation (Figure 4).

Correct: Sit at the head end to initiate BVM ventilation.

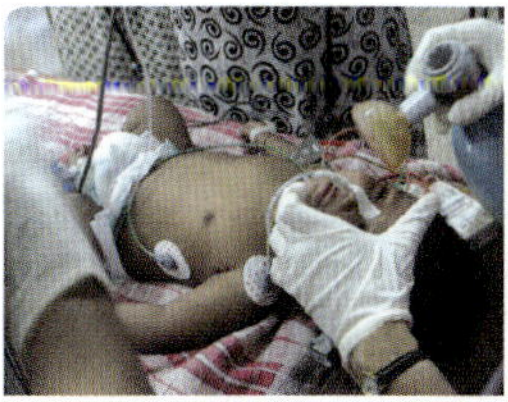

Figure 4: Head tilt, chin lift maneuver performed concurrently with the EC clamp is essential for successful mask ventilation.

Wrong: Standing can compromise the airway by kinking the neck.

Correct:

- The thenar eminence is placed over the forehead to perform the head tilt maneuver.
- The hand is used to clasp the face.
- The trolley is used to support one's elbow.
- The C-clamp is provided by using the thumb and index finger (2 fingers) to encircle the mask *along its rim*. Effort is taken to prevent air leak at the site of exit of the naso-gastric tube (NGT) (Figure 5).

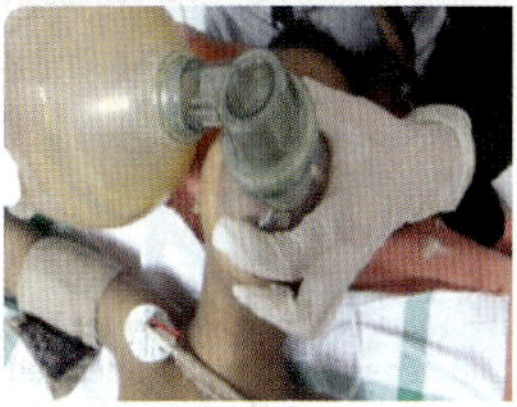

Figure 5: The C-clamp is provided by encircling the rim of the mask with the thumb and index finger.

Wrong: Encircling the top of the mask and pressing it down.

Correct:

- The E clamp is provided by the **m**iddle finger is at the **m**entum, the **r**ing finger at the **r**amus and the **l**ittle finger at the **a**ngle of the jaw (3 fingers) (Figure 6).

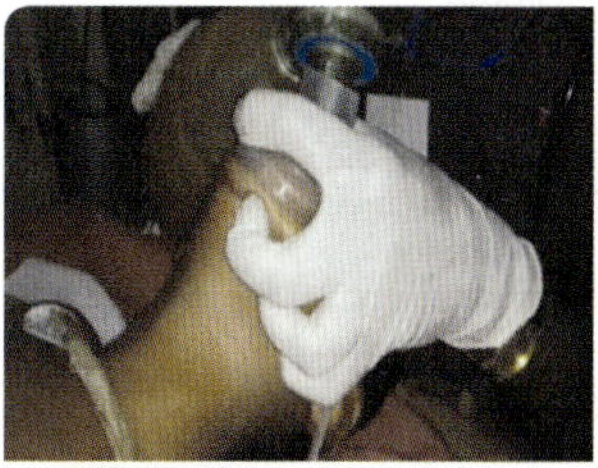

Figure 6: E clamp is provided by middle finger at mentum, ring finger at ramus and little finger at angle of mandible

- Fingers providing E-clamp should be flexed at the all the metaphalangeal joints and used as a hook to lift the jaw (like a bucket handle).

Wrong:

- Bunching fingers used to provide the E-clamp.
- Compression of the soft tissue in the midline thereby worsening airway obstruction.

Effective BVM technique is an art that must be practiced regularly. Effective bag valve mask ventilation is key to neurological intact survival.

ENDOTRACHEAL INTUBATION (FIGURES 11 TO 13)

It is a procedure in which a tube is placed in the trachea to ventilate a child. This skill needs practice. One should master bag mask ventilation technique before learning intubation.

Indications

- Cardiac arrest
- Respiratory failure
- Hypotensive shock
- Signs of pulmonary edema during fluid resuscitation
- Raised intracranial pressure (ICP)
- Low Glasgow coma scale <8 to secure the airway
- Transporting a very sick child.

Equipment Needed for Intubation

SOAP ME is a pneumonic used to prepare oneself prior to intubation.

- **S**-Suction device; both vacuum suction and electrical suction apparatus should be available. Suction catheters both Yankauer and flexible catheters are needed.
- **O**-Oxygen either from a wall source or cylinder. Check the oxygen source before intubation.
- **A**-Airway devices: Age appropriate endo tracheal tubes.
    1. Age appropriate endo tracheal tubes.
    2. Bag valve mask device with reservoir and an appropriate sized mask.
    3. Jackson-Rees circuit
    4. Laryngoscope with curved blade (> 2 years) or straight blade (< 2 years of age).

Bag valve mask device with reservoir and an appropriate sized mask.

1. Jackson-Rees circuit
2. Laryngoscope with curved or straight blade depending upon the age.
3. Check the bulb and battery (Figure 7).
4. Tincture benzoin soaked cotton (used to help dynaplast to stick on to the skin).

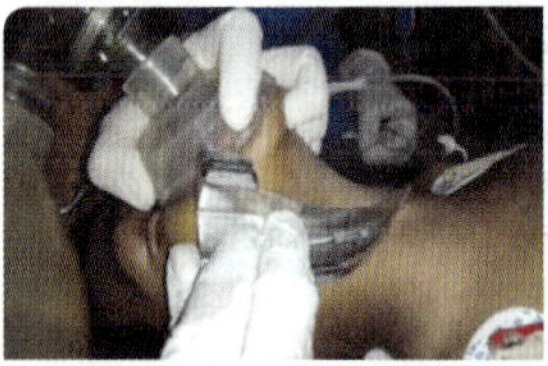

Figure 7: Blade, extending beyond Adam's apple or too short should not be used.

5. Adhesive tapes
6. Nasogastric tubes

- **P**-Pharmacology: Midazolam (0.2 mg/kg) may be used to intubate.

Personnel: Intubation requires a team. The team includes a minimum of 3–4 persons.

1. The airway manager who will intubate
2. Airway nurse: One nurse to suction and assist in intubation.
3. One nurse to suction, assist in intubation and administer midazolam.
4. One doctor to keep track of the pulse oximeter, perform the rapid cardiopulmonary cerebral assessment after intubation and document the procedure.

- **ME**—Monitoring Equipment

Pulse oximeter, cardiac monitor with noninvasive BP are connected to monitor the child during intubation.

Procedure

- Wear gloves and take universal precautions.
- Position the airway with a head tilt and chin lift. If trauma is suspected use the jaw thrust maneuver.
- Insert a nasogastric tube and decompress the stomach. Keep the nasogastric tube open.
- If child is spontaneously breathing preoxygenate using a flow inflating ventilation device.
- If respiratory efforts are inadequate or child is hypoxic start ventilation with bag valve mask.
- It is preferable to have 2 vascular lines one for giving fluids/inotropes and the other to administer medications to induce sedation.
- Cricoid pressure (Sellick's maneuver) is applied soon after the sedatives and analgesics are given. This helps to facilitate a good view of the glottis (Figure 8).
- As soon as the anesthetic drugs have been administered, layers of pads are placed beneath the shoulders to help align the oropharynx with the laryngopharynx. The external auditory meatus, should be aligned with the anterior aspect of the shoulder.
- Pre-oxygenate, until saturations are 100%. The duration of pre-oxygenation may be titrated based on the severity of illness.
- This helps to prevent desaturation during intubation.

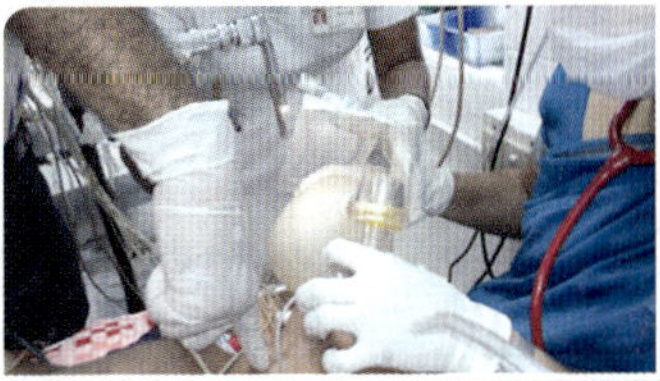

Figure 8: Sellick's maneuver during bag valve mask ventilation. The airway nurse is holding the laryngoscope and the tube in a position accessible for the airway manager.

- Hold the handle of the laryngoscope in the left hand and insert the blade into the mouth. The tip of the blade is placed in the vallecula (the space between the base of the tongue and the epiglottis). The blade is used to sweep the tongue to the left. In infants, the straight blade is used to lift the epiglottis and visualize the glottis (Figures 9 and 13).

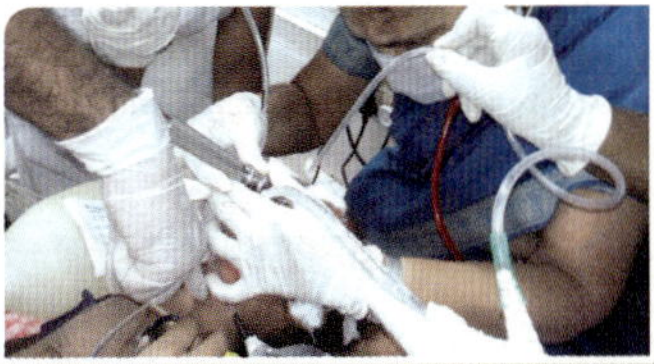

Figure 9: Insert laryngoscope only up to tip of epiglottis. Note the need for two suction tips: Yankauer and suction catheter.

- After the blade is properly positioned, exert upward traction in the direction of the long axis of the handle to expose the glottis.

- Insert the endotracheal tube (ET) from the right corner of the mouth into the glottis under direct visualization. The vocal cord mark is a dark line in the endotracheal tube (Figure 14). When the tube is inserted until this mark, it ensures that the tip of the tube is in the trachea.
- Cuffed tracheal tubes are inserted until the cuff is positioned just below the vocal cords.
- Intubation attempt should not exceed 10 seconds.
- Prolonged attempts can cause hypoxia and bradycardia.
- Stop the procedure if child deteriorates and ventilate with a BVM till saturation improves to 100%. Suction the airway if needed.
- Once the tube is in place, confirm tube position by 5-point auscultation.
- Auscultate both infraclavicular and axillary areas and in the epigastric region.
- Apply tincture benzoin to the skin and secure the tube in position using dynaplast (Figures 10 and 11).

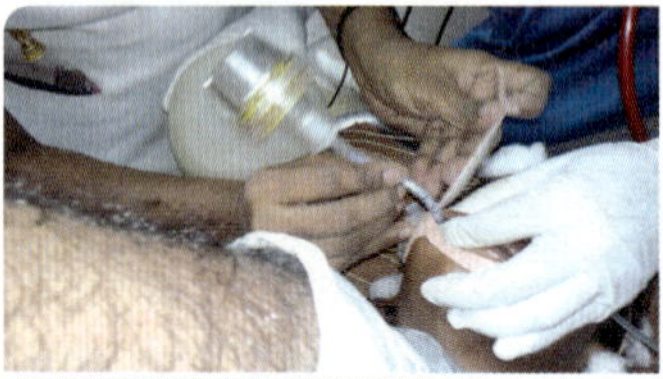

Figure 10: Intubation is not complete until tube is fixed securely.

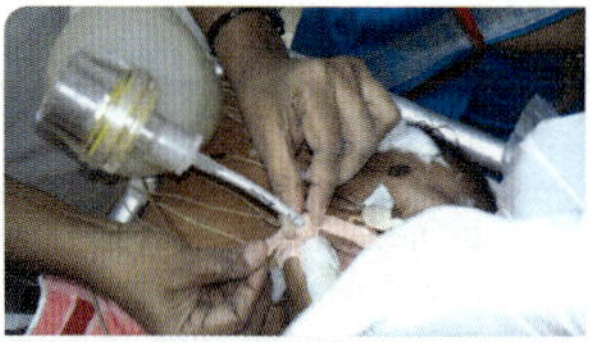

Figure 11: Note 2 strips of dynaplast are needed to secure the ET tube

- Before the ET is taped in place once again check correct position by 5 point auscultation (Figure 12).

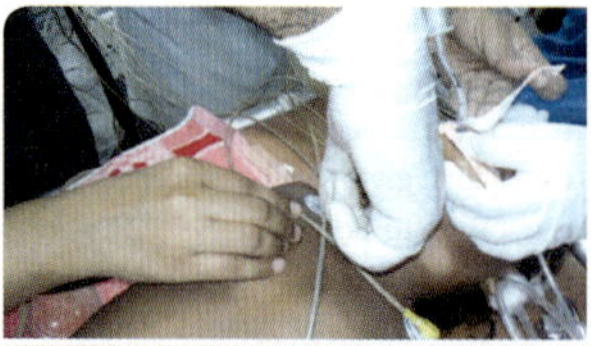

Figure 12: Right infra-clavicular followed by left, right infra-axillary, left infra-axillary followed by epigastric region.

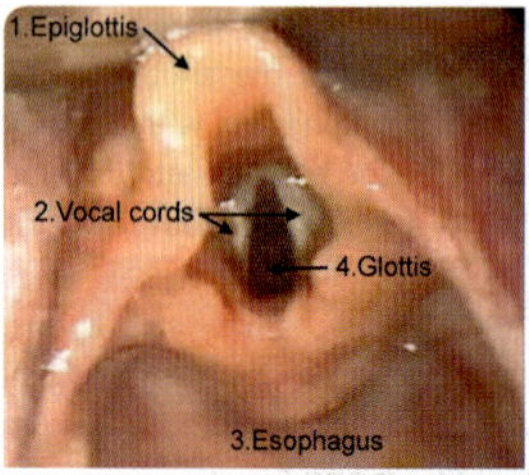

Figure 13: View of the cords during laryngoscopy.

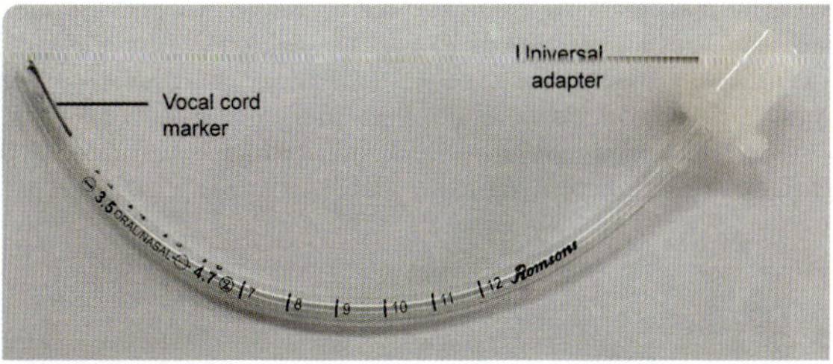

Figure 14: Endotracheal tube.

- Perform cardiopulmonary cerebral assessment and document (Figure 10).
- Document the procedure in detail including how many attempts have been made, any complication observed, size of the tube, drugs used. The distance marker at the lips should be noted to identify any accidental tube displacement.

Complications

- Local trauma to mouth and oropharynx
- Airway edema and subglottic stenosis
- Hypoxia, bradycardia and cardiac arrest during procedure.

Note:

1. If in doubt that tube is not in the correct place, take it out and initiate bag valve mask ventilation.
2. If air entry is reduced on the left side, suspect right main bronchus intubation. Slowly withdraw endotracheal tube until air entry is equal and infiate bag valve mark ventilation.
3. Consider DOPE (displacement, obstruction, pneumothorax, equipment failure) when a ventilated child deterio-rates.

Common Errors

1. Hyperextension of the neck can obscure the view of the cords
2. Not placing a pad of cloth under the shoulders or under the head
3. Not checking the light source, bag and mask and battery before intubation.

LARYNGEAL MASK AIRWAY (LMA)

Introduction

It is not uncommon to feel panic when encountering an apneic child in pre-hospital settings. Lack of team support, anxious parents and lack of skills can delay provision of ventilation to the seriously ill child.

The laryngeal mask airway is a bridge between intubation and bag valve mask ventilation.

- Its major advantage is its ease of insertion (as easy as insertion of an orogastric tube).

- Inflation of the mask following insertion seals the esophagus and permits air to enter exclusively into the trachea.

The LMA is a small inflatable mask, attached to tubing with a universal adapter. It is designed to sit in the oropharynx with the tip in the hypopharynx and the base at the epiglottis. With the cuff inflated, the laryngeal mask creates a seal around the supra-glottic area, allowing air flow between the tubing and trachea (Figures 15A and B)

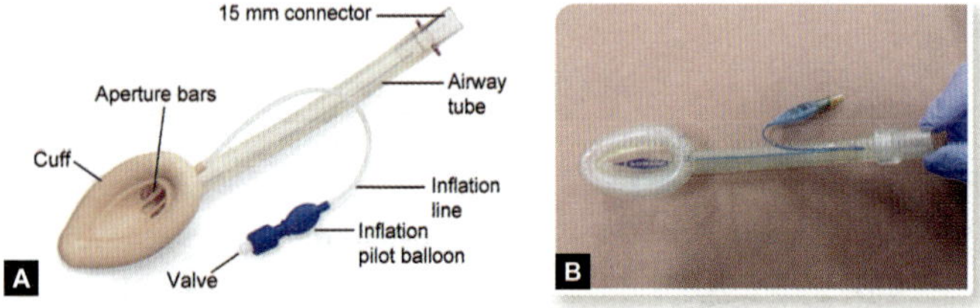

Figures 15A and B: (A) Parts of the laryngeal mask airway (LMA); (B) Parts of the laryngeal mask airway (LMA).

- Place an inflation syringe in the cuff valve and deflate the cuff completely before insertion, making sure that the leading tip is not folded backward (Figure 16).
- Lubricate the posterior surface of the LMA with a water soluble lubricant (Figure 17).

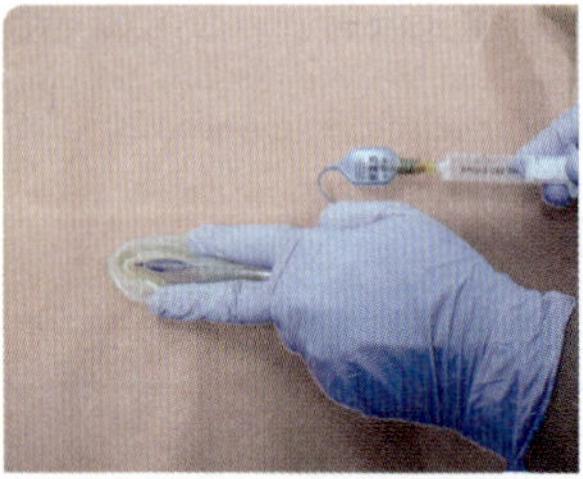

Figure 16: Deflation of laryngeal mask cuff.

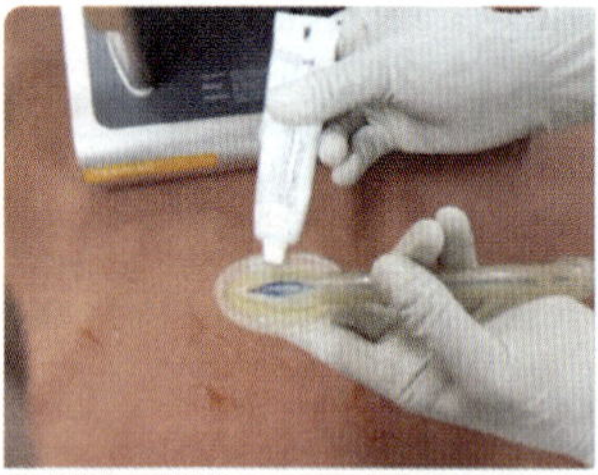

Figure 17: Application of jelly prior to insertion.

Lubrication of the posterior surface of the LMA permits it to slide easily. Lubrication of the larygneal opening should be avoided. Curling of the mask should also be avoided, since it can cause occlusion of the glottis by the epiglottis.

- Hold the LMA close to the cuff using a pencil grip (Figure 18).

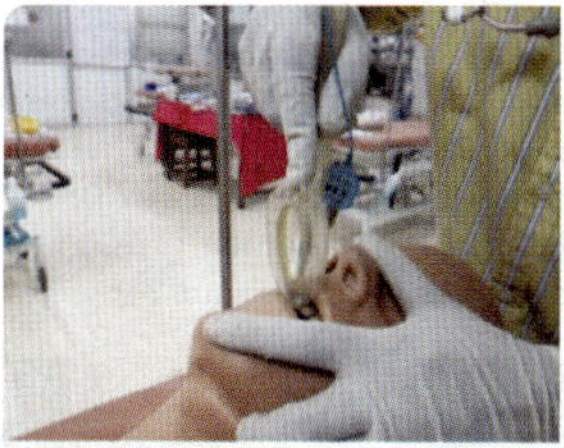

Figure 18: Hold the LMA at the junction of the mask and the tube using a pencil grip.

- Place the head and neck in the sniffing position. Open the mouth, while lifting the chin forward (Figure 19).

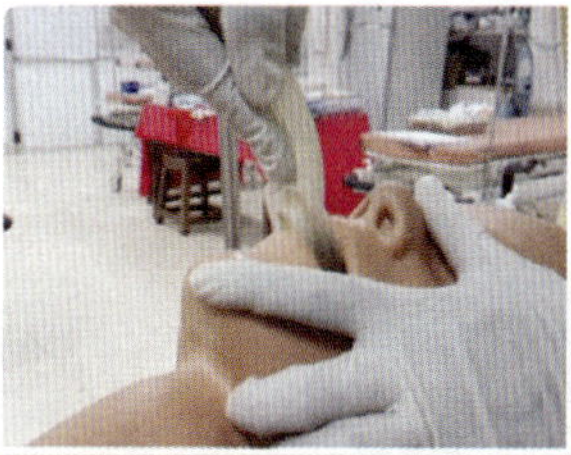

Figure 19: Insert the LMA, by pushing the mask along the hard palate in the mid-line.

- To facilitate LMA introduction into the oral cavity, gently press the middle finger down on the jaw.
- Simultaneously, press the LMA against the hard palate and guide it along the posterior oropharynx until the operator feels firm resistance. The opening of the cuff faces towards the tongue. This method prevents folding up of the epiglottis (Figure 20).

Maintaining pressure with the finger on the tube in the cranial direction, advance the mask until definite resistance is felt at the base of the hypopharynx. Note the flexion of the wrist (Figure 20).

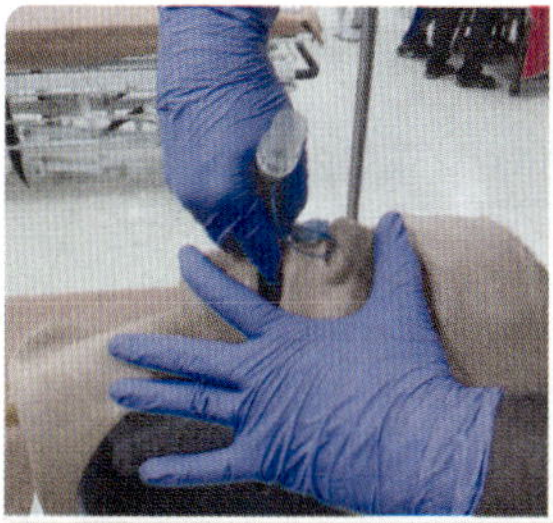

Figure 20: Index finger is used to push the laryngeal mask along the hard palate.

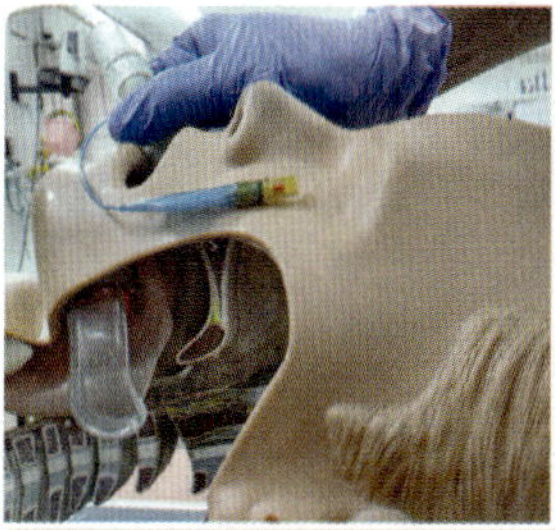

Figure 21: Mannequin showing the final position of the Laryngeal mask airway (LMA) over the glottis.

Through out the insertion, take steps to avoid getting bitten by the victim. The LMA, can be inserted only if the victim is completely unconscious.

- Inflate the cuff using an air filled syringe until the pilot balloon gets filled up. The laryngeal mask may be observed to 'rise up' slightly out of the oropharynx (Figures 21, 22A and B).
- Fix the LMA in the midline with dynaplast tape around the tube. Also insert a roll of gauze on either side of the LMA to avoid biting the tube (Figure 23).
- Prior to removal of the LMA, the pilot balloon is deflated (Figure 24).

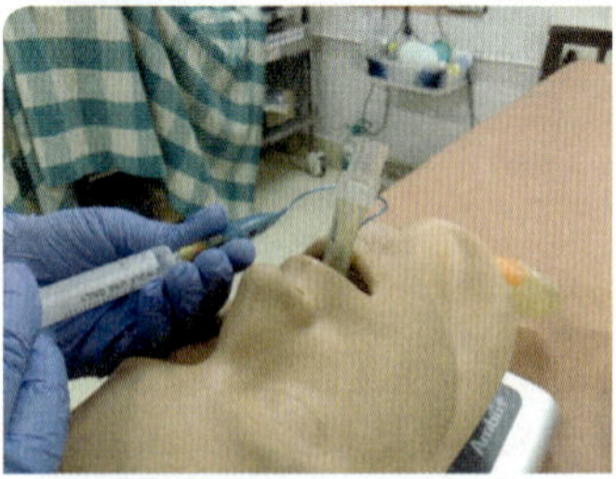

Figure 22A: Inflating the mask by pushing air.

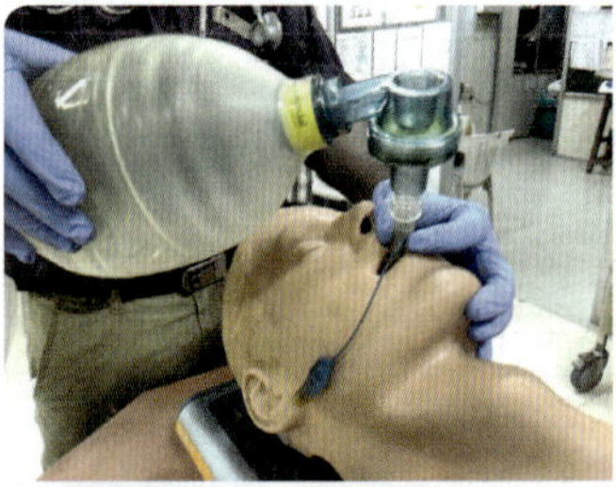

Figure 22B: Connecting the bag valve mask to the Laryngeal mask airway (LMA).

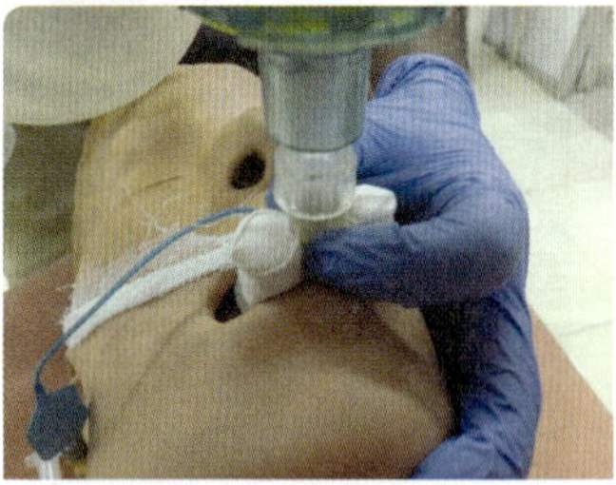

Figure 23: Securing the laryngeal mask airway LMA.

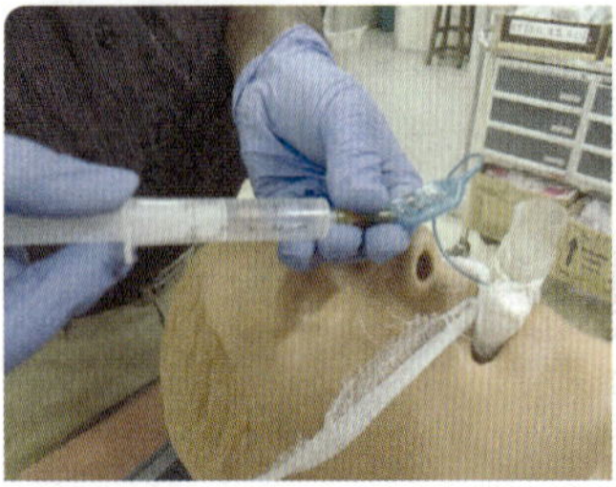

Figure 24: Deflation of laryngeal mask using a syringe, prior to removal of Laryngeal mask airway LMA

BREATHING SPONTANEOUSLY

NON-REBREATHING MASK (FIGURE 25)

Non-rebreathing mask helps to administer 80–90% FiO_2 and is useful in children with effortless tachypnea and shock.

The one way valve between the reservoir and the mask ensures a high concentration of oxygen is inhaled. The one way valve on the side of the mask aid in passage of exhaled tidal volume into the atmosphere. It cannot re-enter the reservoir.

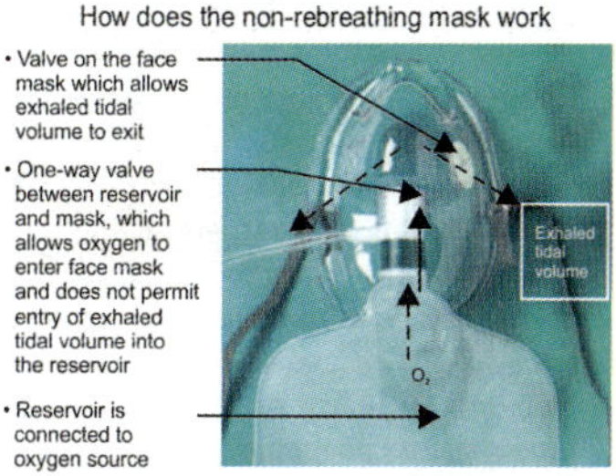

Figure 25: The parts of the non-rebreathing mask and how each part helps to provide nearly 90% FiO_2.

FLOW INFLATING VENTILATION DEVICE (FIGURE 26)

The flow inflating ventilation device (Jackson-Rees circuit or the Bain's circuit), as it is commonly known, is useful in a wide variety of respiratory conditions in seriously ill children. Its major advantage lies in the fact that it provides continuous positive airway pressure in addition to 100% oxygen.

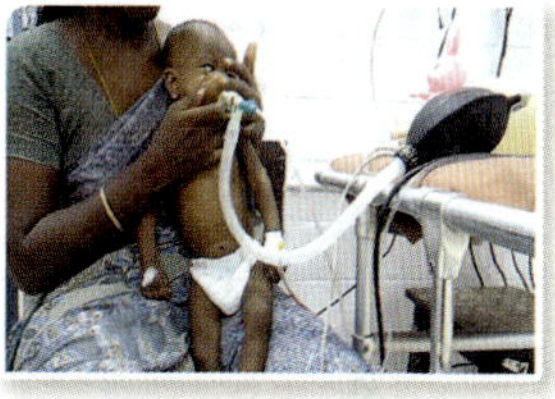

Figure 26: Mother can hold the mask and provide oxygen in this infant with respiratory distress in a non-threatening manner.

PARTS OF THE FLOW INFLATING VENTILATION DEVICE (FIGURE 27)

HOW CPAP HELPS:

- Continuous positive pressure ventilation (CPAP) keeps the upper airway open by opposing the forces that cause dynamic airway collapse.
- CPAP is also useful in children presenting with respiratory failure due to chronic upper airway obstruction:
  a. Laryngomalacia
  b. Abductor nerve palsy
- CPAP aids in opening up the airways that are closed due to bronchospasm or bronchiolitis, especially during expiration.

  CPAP, thereby helps to tide over, impending respiratory failure due to asthma or bronchiolitis whilst the primary disease is being treated.
- In addition, it opens up to collapsed alveoli, thus improving alveolar recruitment and oxygenation in children with pneumonia or pulmonary edema.

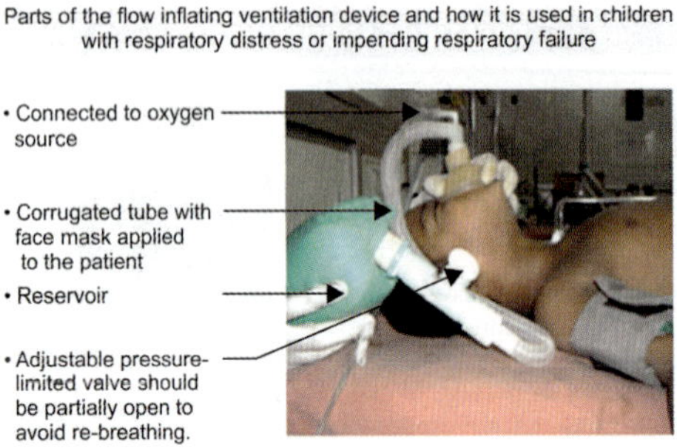

Figure 27: Parts of the flow inflating ventilation device and how it is used.

- Decreases work of breathing.
  The respiratory muscles become tired when children have respiratory distress. CPAP helps to reduce the work of breathing thereby preventing deterioration to respiratory arrest.
- CPAP reduces after-load and pre-load to the failing heart thereby increasing cardiac output. The latter results in improvement in pulmonary congestion (Figure 28).
- The Jackson Rees circuit, helps to provide CPAP for children presenting with respiratory distress or failure due to cardiogenic and non-cardiogenic pulmonary edema secondary to severe sepsis, submersion injury, scorpion envenomation, status epilepticus.

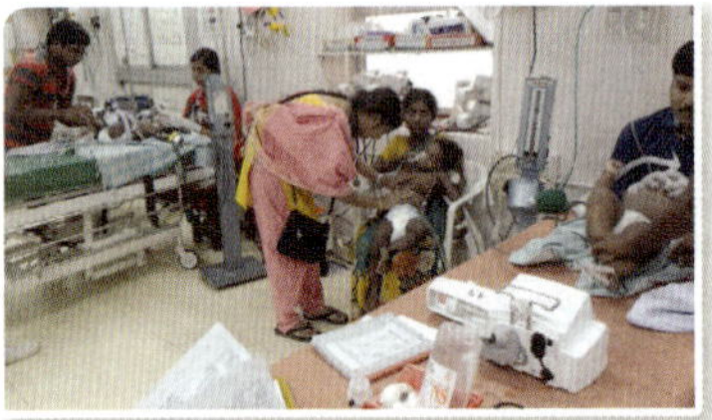

Fig. 28: This picture shows how the Jackson Rees circuit is being used to provides 100% Oxygen with CPAP during resuscitation for pulmonary edema and shock in a busy pediatric emergency department.

KEY POINTS

1. Prior to bag valve mask ventilation, perform head tilt chin lift maneuver, suction oro-pharynx and decompress stomach.
2. Use LMA in unresponsive victims
3. Jackson Rees circuit is useful in children presenting with respiratory distress.

3 CHAPTER

Cardiac Arrest

Chapter Outline

- Basic life support (BLS)
- How to perform good quality chest compression?
- How to use the automated external defibrillator?

BASIC LIFE SUPPORT (BLS)

If a child or infant appears unconscious, check for responsiveness after ruling out that the environment is safe. (No whizzing cars, fire, etc.)

CHECK FOR RESPONSIVENESS

- Older child: Tap the shoulder and shout, "are you ok?" (Figure 1)

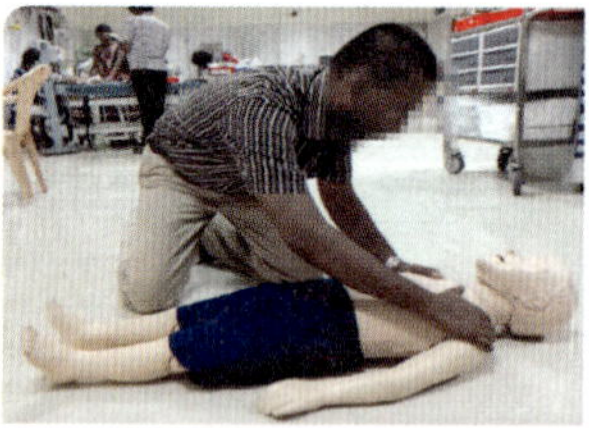

Figure 1: Are you OK?

- Infant: Flick the bottom of the foot to check for unresponsiveness (Figure 2).

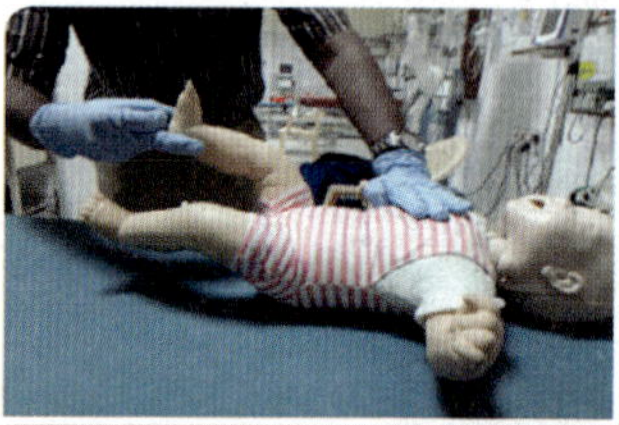

Figure 2: Flick sole to check responsiveness of infant.

IF CHILD/INFANT RESPONDS

- Place on back and open the airway using head tilt chin lift maneuver (Figure 2)
- Ask questions to find out what happened
- Call 108

- Perform a rapid head to toe examination.

IF NOT RESPONSIVE

Airway

- Open airway using head tilt chin lift maneuver (Figures 3 and 4)

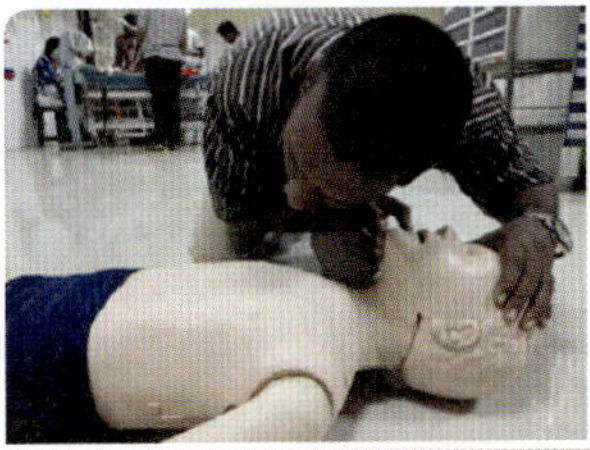

Figure 3: Assessment of breathing in a child.

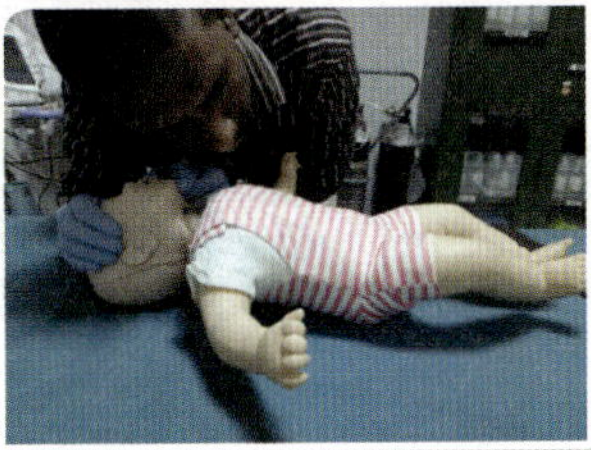

Figure 4: Assessment of breathing in a child.

Breathing

- Check for breathing (Do not check for more than 10 seconds) (Figures 3 and 4)
- If not breathing or jaw breathing, initiate mouth to mouth or mouth to mask ventilation
- Give 2 rescue breaths
- Child: Pinch the nose shut, then make a complete seal over child's mouth (Figure 5)

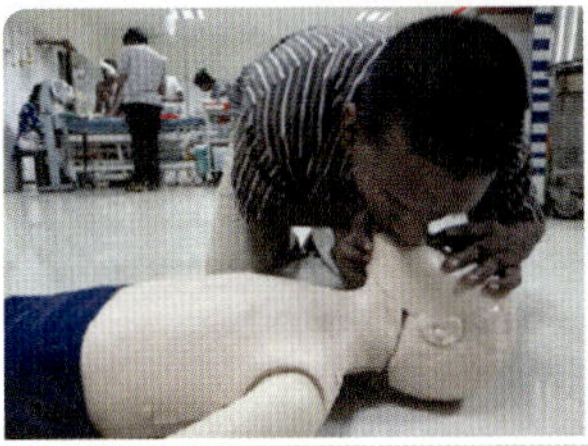

Figure 5: Pinch nose. Seal mouth with rescuer's mouth and blow air.

- Infant: Make complete seal over infant's mouth and nose (Figure 6).

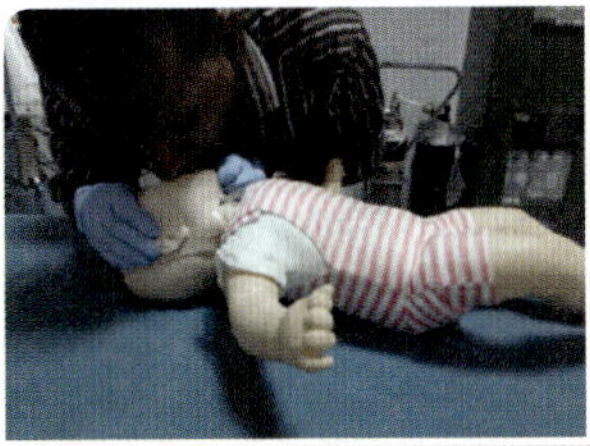

Figure 6: Make a seal of nose and mouth and give breath.

- Blow in for about 1 second to make the chest clearly rise.
- Give 2 rescue breaths, one after the other

- If the chest does not rise with rescue breaths, re-tilt the head and blow once more (rescue breath)
- After providing 2 rescue breaths, start chest compression (discussed later).

UNCONSCIOUS FOLLOWING CHOKING: CHILD AND INFANT

- Chest does not rise with rescue breaths
- Re-tilt head and give rescue breaths
- Give 30 chest compressions
- Look for and remove foreign body if seen
- Avoid blind finger sweep
- Continue cycles of CPR. Do not stop CPR unless the child starts breathing, you are exhausted or environment is un-safe.

CHOKING

What Should I do If A Child is Choking and Conscious?

Choking is characterized by not being able to cough, speak or breathe.

- Stand or kneel behind the child, depending on his or her size

Abdominal Thrusts (Figure 7)

- Make a fist with the thumb side of your hand above the umbilicus in the middle of the abdomen.
- Cover your fist with your other hand.
- Give 5 rapid upward abdominal thrusts.

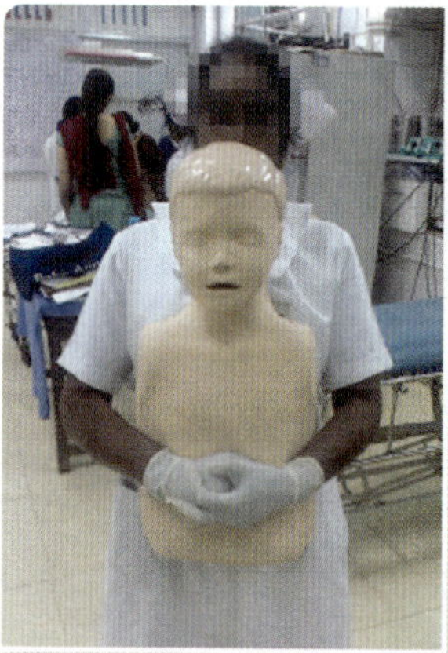

Figure 7: Abdominal thrust.

CONTINUE ABDOMINAL THRUSTS UNTIL

The foreign body is:

- Coughed out and can breathe or
- Child becomes unresponsive.

The first aid maneuver that is used to expel foreign in a choking episode is called Heimlich maneuver.

How does the Heimlich's maneuver work?
It is a technique wherein abdominal thrusts are used to lift the diaphragm and expel air from the lungs, thereby causing the foreign object to be expelled from the airway.

Conscious Choking Infant (Figure 8)

The infant is not able to cough, cry or breathe.

- Sit at the edge of a chair such that your knee is below your hip.
- Support the infant on your left arm with the infant's head placed face down. The arm holding the infant is supported on your left knee

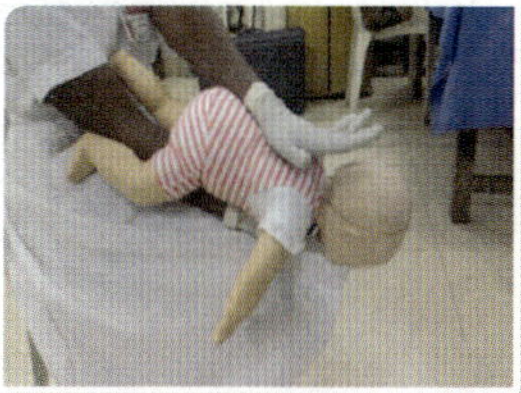

Figure 8: Choking infant who is conscious: Back blows.

5 BACK BLOWS

- With the heel of the right hand, hit 5 times between the infant's shoulder blades.

CHEST THRUSTS (FIGURE 9)

- Turn the baby on the right arm and right knee, face up
- Place two or three fingers in the center of the infant's chest just below the nipple line and press the sternum for about 1½ inches.
- Examine oral cavity and remove the foreign body if visualized.
- Avoid blind finger sweep

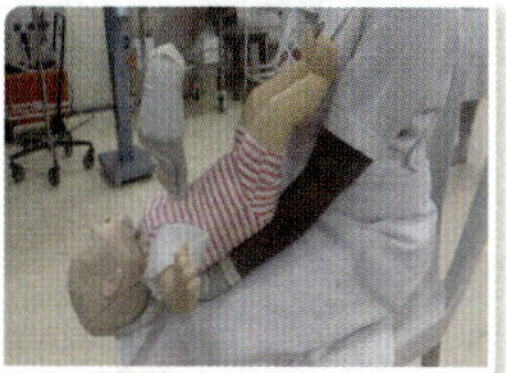

Figure 9: Choking infant who is conscious: Chest thrust.

If Foreign Body is not Visualized Repeat Back Blows and Chest Thrusts

- Repeat until the foreign body is coughed out.
- Child can breathe
- Child becomes un-responsive

If the Child Becomes Unresponsive/ Unconscious During Choke Relief Maneuver

1. Make the child lie down in firm surface
2. Initiate chest compressions
3. Just before delivering assisted breath, open the mouth and try visualize the foreign body
4. If visualized, remove carefully
   If not, continue chest compressions and ventilation till help arrives.

HOW TO USE THE DEFIBRILLATOR

A defibrillator is a device that delivers a high energy electric shock to the heart through the chest wall to someone who is in cardiac arrest due to ventriculr tachycardia of fibrillation.

The device is equipped with 2 paddles that are used to deliver the shock (Figure 11). Pulseless electrical activity or asystole are more common than VF/VT in children wherein, immediate, bag valve mask

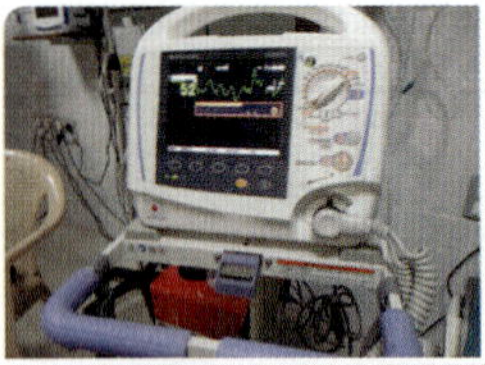

Figure 10: Defibrillator

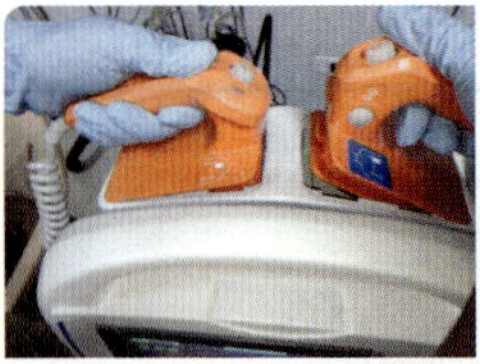

Figure 11: Paddles, are placed on the top of the defibrillator.

ventilation and chest compression is mandatory. (Searching for a defibrillator, will not improve the outcomes in asystole or pulseless electrical activity).

Some machines have smaller paddles (child size) within the adult paddles (Figures 12 to 14).

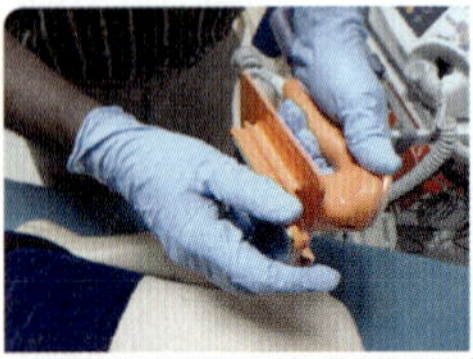

Figure 12: Pediatric paddles are placed within the adult paddles.

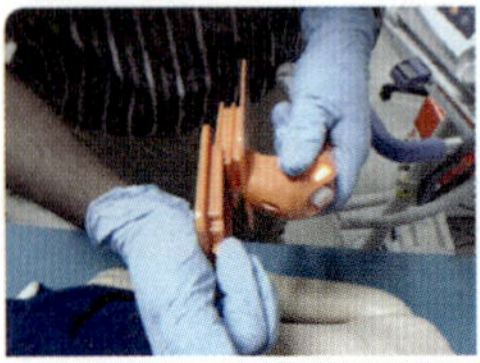

Figure 13: Pediatric paddles can be slipped from the adult paddles when needed.

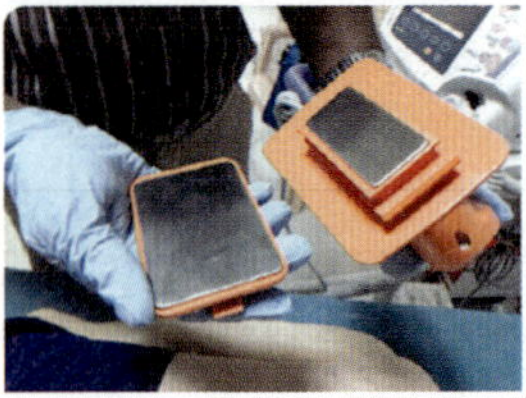

Figure 14: The adult paddle and the child paddle are now separate.

Defibrillation: The electrical shock is not timed with the heart's electrical cycle.

Defibrillation is performed only when Shockable rhythms are noted:

- Pulseless ventricular tachycardia
- Ventricular fibrillation.

Cardioversion is performed for the following:

- Ventricular tachycardia with pulse
- Supraventricular tachycardia
- Atrial fibrillation
- Atrial flutter

How to Use the Defibrillator

- Step 1: Turn on the machine.

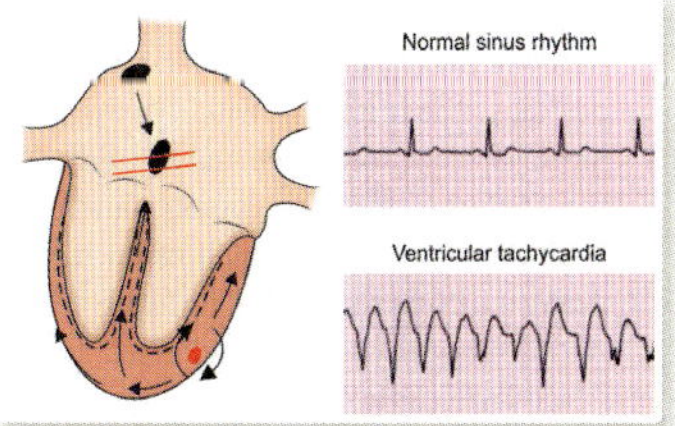

Figure 15: VT occurs due to the disorganized electrical activity of the purkinje fibers in comparison to the normal electrophysiology of the heart.

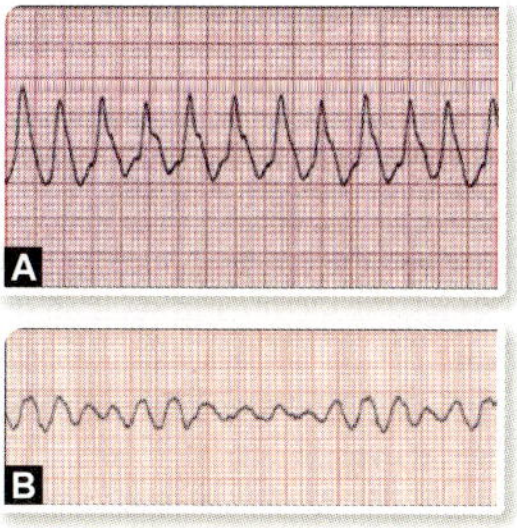

Figures 16A and B: Note the broad complex QRS complexes characteristic of VT.

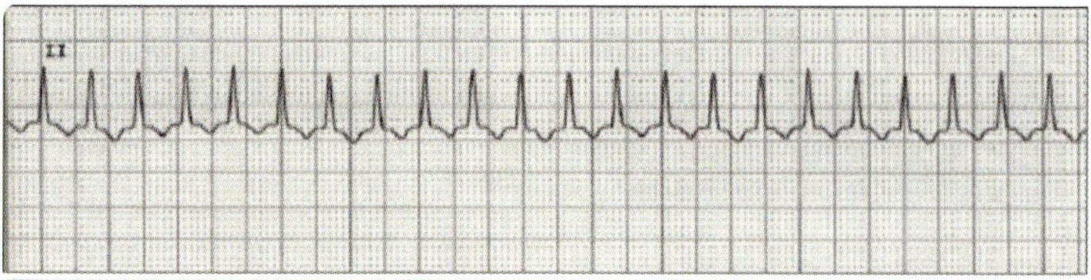

Figure 16C: Ventricular tachycardia

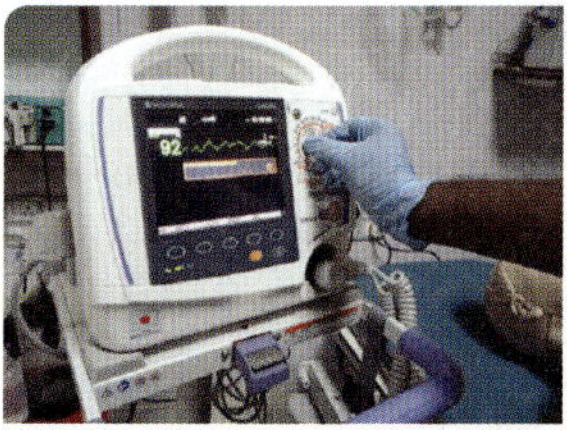

Figure 17: Step 1: Set the calculated energy (Joules/kg) by turning the knob on the machine.

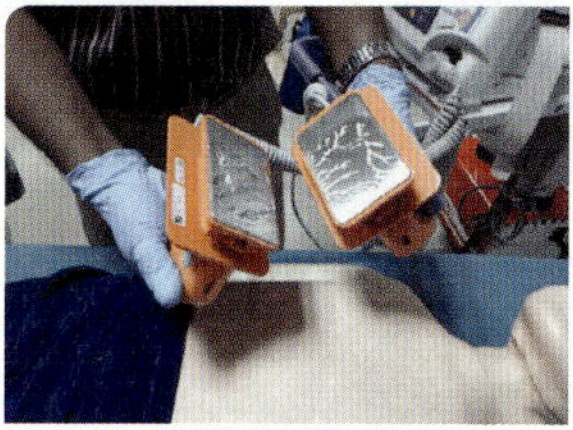

Figure 18: Step 2: Apply jelly to the paddles.

If child has supra-ventricular tachycardia, turn on the synchronized mode. If, child has ventricular tachycardia or ventricular fibrillation, this step is not needed.

Calculate the dose (joules/kg) needed to shock the victim and set it on the machine

- Step 2: Apply jelly on to the paddles and smear it evenly

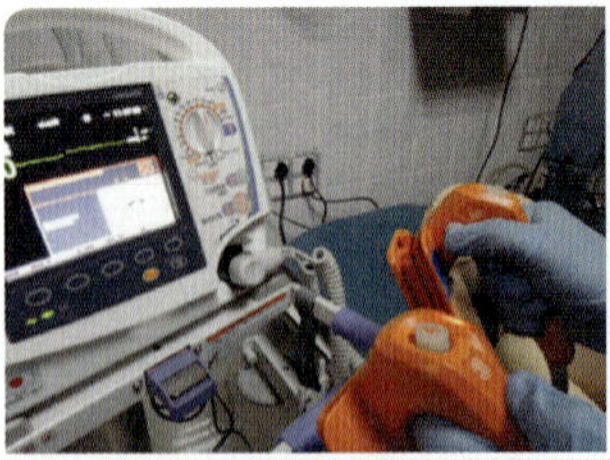

Figure 19: Step 3: Charge by pressing the charge button on the paddle.

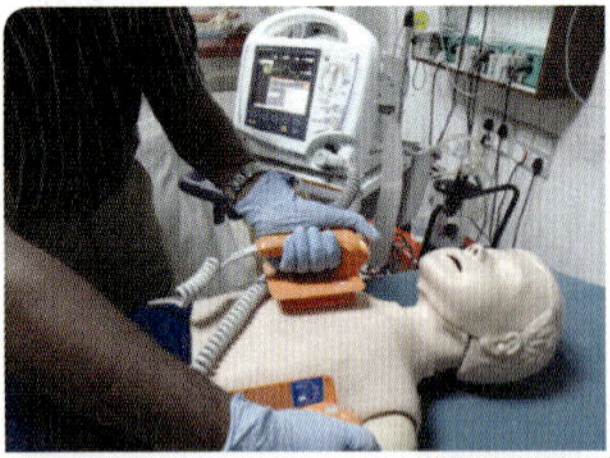

Figure 21: Step 5: Discharge electrical charge (defibrillate). Note the thumbs on both hands pressing the discharge buttons on the paddles.

- Step 3: Charge the paddles by simultaneously pressing the button on both the paddles. The indicator will light up.
- Step 4: Place one (sternal) paddle on the sternum and one (apex) paddle on the apex. The paddles will often have a picture or text that helps indicate which paddle should be placed where.

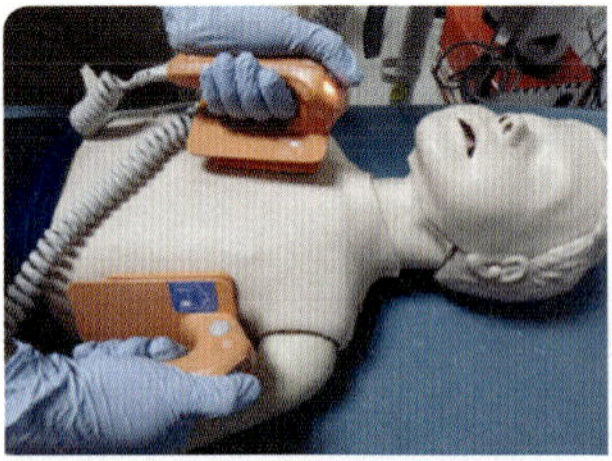

Figure 20: Step 4: Place paddles, one on the sternum and one on the apex. Call out "I clear, you clear, Oxygen clear (turn of oxygen). All personnel stand clear of the metal parts of the trolley.

- *While performing Defibrillation followed by CPR, consider and correct reversible causes of cardiac arrest (4Hs and 4Ts):*
- *Hypoxia*
- *Hypovolemia*
- *Hyper/hypokalemia, metabolic*
- *Hypothermia*
- *Thromboembolism (coronary or pulmonary)*
- *Tension pneumothorax*
- *Tamponade (cardiac)*
- *Toxic/therapeutic disturbance*

Call out: I am clear, you are clear, oxygen clear (disconnect oxygen) if the child is being ventilated

- Step 5: Discharge, by pressing the appropriate button on the paddle
- Step 6 (not shown): Immediately after shock application, continue CPR as per PALS guidelines.

HOW TO PERFORM GOOD QUALITY CHEST COMPRESSION

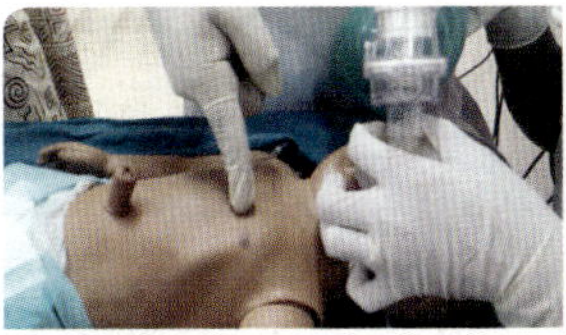

Figure 22: Location of chest compression is one finger breadth below the line drawn between the nipples.

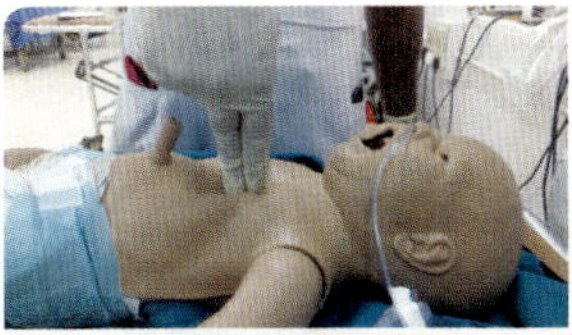

Figure 23: Infant CPR in out of hospital settings, where if you are the only rescuer, 2 fingers may be used as shown to provide chest compressions.

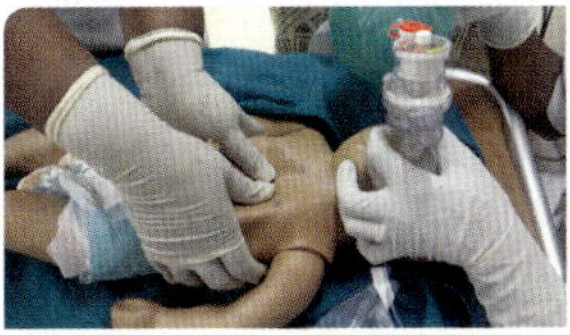

Figure 24: Clasp the chest and apply pressure by approximating thumbs if you have one more rescuer.

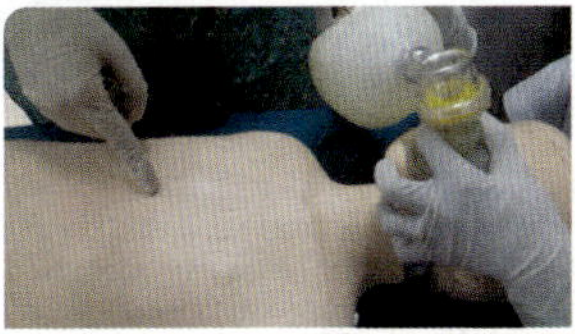

Figure 25: Draw line along the right costal margin.

- *If you are alone (single rescuer), perform five cycles of compressions and breaths on the child (two minutes) and call for help.*

Use two hands (one on top the other), or heel of one hand if the child is very small, to perform chest compressions. Press straight down on (approximately 5 cms). If the child is an adolescent, push straight down on the chest at least 6 cms.

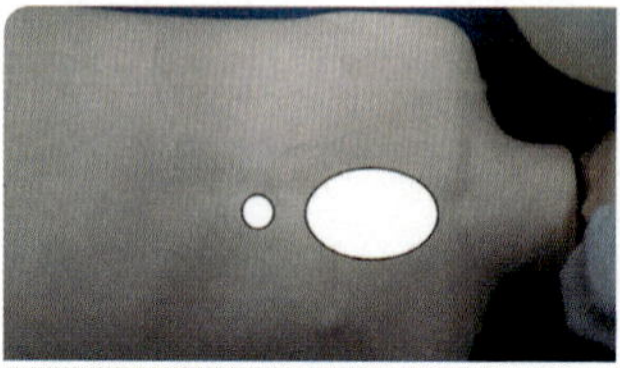

Figure 26: Avoid xiphoid and use the center of the sternum to provide chest compressions.

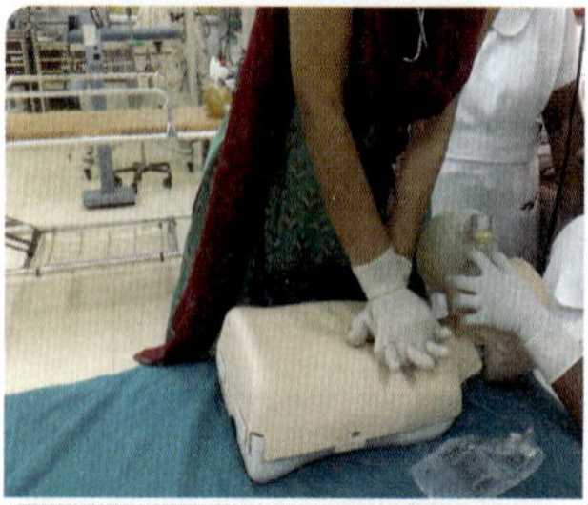

Figure 28: Two hand technique is used in children beyond 8 years of age. Fingers are interlocked and the second hand is used to extend the first and apply greater pressure.

Draw a line along the costal margin. Identify the xiphoid process.

Clinically, the xiphoid process plays an important role as a bony anatomical landmark in the trunk. It can be damaged by improperly administered CPR, leading to injury to the underlying organs.

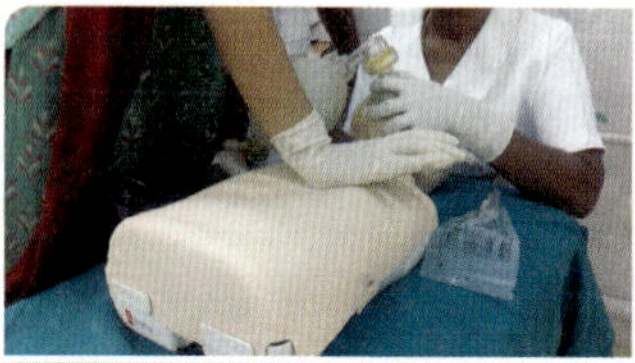

Figure 27: Child CPR. The heel of one hand is used to apply chest compression in the child between 1–8 years. The wrist is extended to ensure correct position. The elbows must be straight. The rescuer should be directly above the victim.

- *Avoid flexing your elbows during chest compressions (Keep your elbows straight).*
- *Shoulders should be directly above the chest to exert maximum pressure.*
- *Avoid rocking or bending during compressions*
- *Avoid double crossing on hands during chest compressions.*

EPINEPHRINE

As bag valve mask ventilation and chest compressions are in progress, epinephrine is administered (0.1 mL/kg of 1:10,000) intravenously. A bolus of 5 mL of normal saline is administered to flush the medication into the circulation. A dose is given following 2 minutes of CPR. If bradycardic, or hypotensive, an epinephrine infusion is initiated at the rate of 0.3 μg/kg/minute. If IV access is unavailable, the intraosseous route or the intratracheal route may be used. The dose may be increased by 10 times when the intratracheal route is used.

Flowchart 1: Summary of good quality CPR

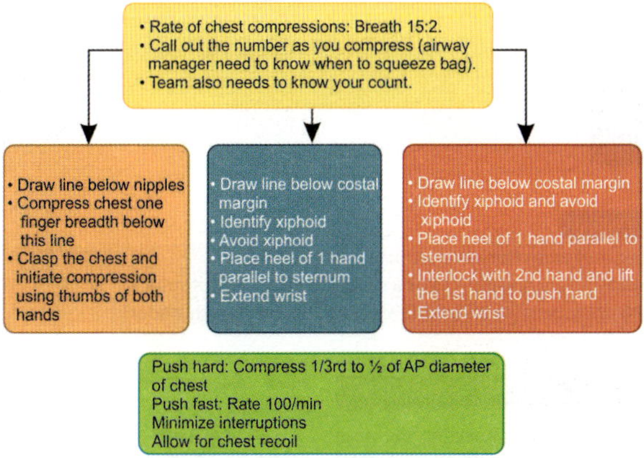

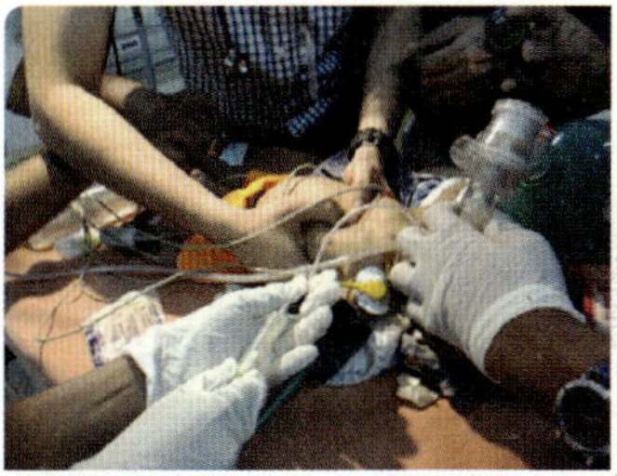

KEY POINTS

1. Hypoxia is the commonest cause of bradycardia in children.
2. Immediate initiation of BVM ventilation is crucial to successful resuscitation
3. Age appropriate chest compression should be provided.
4. Need for defibrillation is not as common in children as in adults

4 CHAPTER

Stridor

Chapter Outline

- Applied anatomy of airway obstruction.
- How to avoid aggravating hypoxia during management of stridor?
- How to assess severity of hypoxia and shock in a child with stridor?

STRIDOR

The airway is a tube connecting the nose to the bronchi. Even minimal mucosal edema can significantly reduce the diameter of the pediatric airway and increase resistance to air flow and work of breathing.

Different parts of the airway are more prone for obstruction than others. Anatomically, the upper airway is divided into (Figure 1):

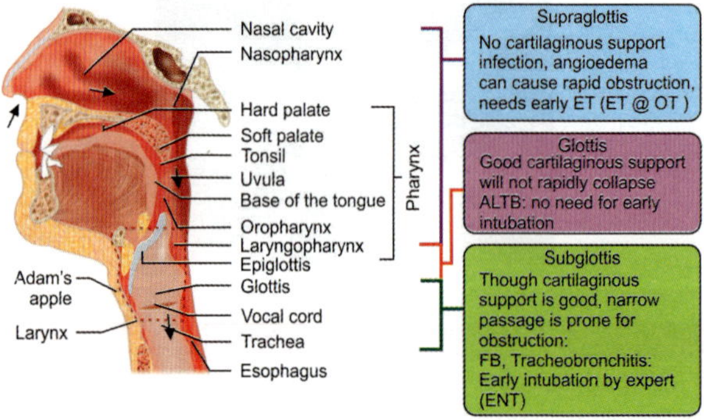

Figure 1: Presentation and etiology varies on the level of obstruction. The anatomical region that becomes obstructed, impacts therapeutic decisions.

- *Supraglottis:* This region is surrounded by soft tissue and has no cartilaginous support. Hence, supraglottic obstruction is prone for complete obstruction.
- *Glottis (vocal cords):* Cartilaginous support protects the airway, thus protecting it from collapsing.
- *Subglottis:* Cartilaginous support is better than the supraglottis region. However, in infants, the supporting cartilage is much less developed and the entire passage is much more narrower than adults.

> *Crying can aggravate hypoxia by increasing air turbulence in the obstructed airway. All precautions should be taken to prevent a child with stridor from crying.*

- **Avoid separating mother and child.**

Examine and manage the child on his mother's lap.

- **Avoid changing the position of comfort which the child has adopted.**

Complete airway obstruction may be precipitated if the child is placed on the trolley for examination or taking an X-ray.

- **Avoid forcing an oxygen mask on a screaming child.**
- **Mother is encouraged to hold the oxygen delivery device in a nonthreatening manner.**

Presentation and etiology varies based on the level of obstruction. The anatomical regions of the airway that is obstructed, impacts therapeutic decisions.

Assessment of stridor based on severity of hypoxia (Figures 2A to D).

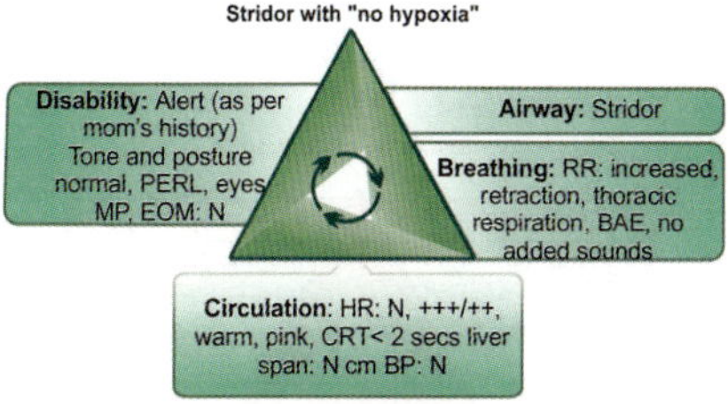

Figure 2A: A: Stridor; **B:** Respiratory distress; **C:** HR (Normal for age), No shock, BP (Normal for age), No cardiac dysfunction; **D:** Nil

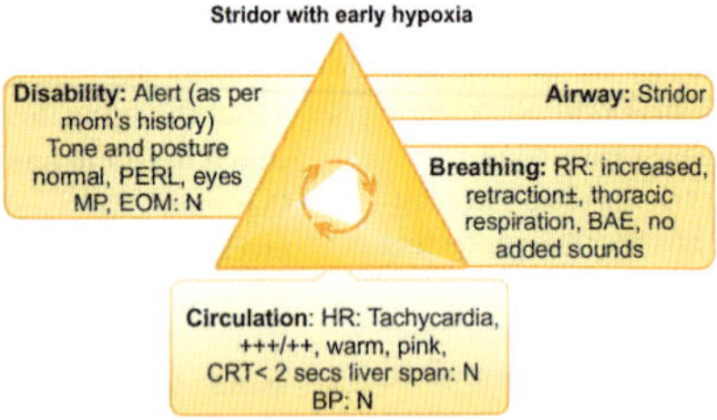

Figure 2B: A: Stridor; **B:** Respiratory distress; **C:** Tachycardia, No shock, no cardiac dysfunction, BP normal for age; **D:** Nil

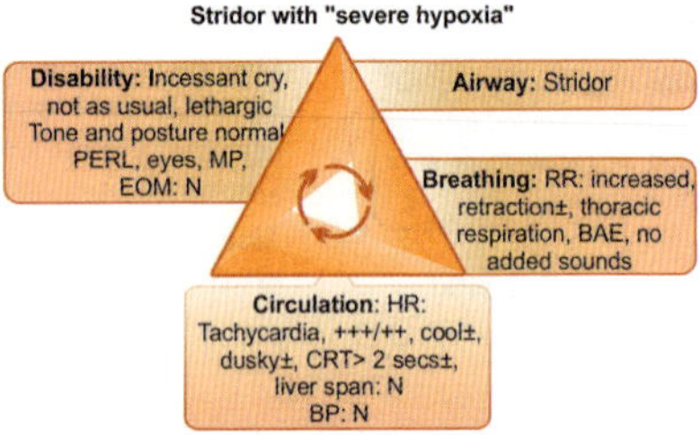

Figure 2C: A: Stridor; **B:** Respiratory distress; **C:** Tachycardia, shock, no cardiac dysfunction, BP normal; **D:** ALOC

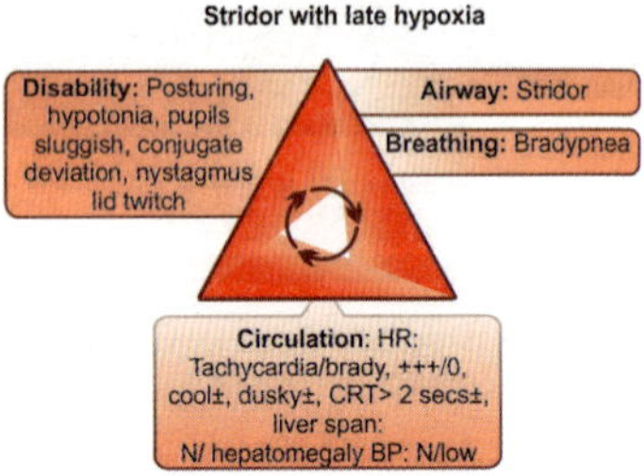

Figure 2D: A: Stridor; **B:** Respiratory failure; **C:** Tachycardia/bradycardia, shock, with cardiac dysfunction, relative hypotension or low BP; **D:** ALOC with non-convulsive status epilepticus.

Management of stridor based on etiology and severity of hypoxia is provided in Table 1.

Early recognition of severity of hypoxia, due to airway obstruction, is based on mother's history of altered mental status and the rapid cardiopulmonary cerebral assessment. The pulse oximeter will pick up hypoxia only when the blood oxygen levels drop to 60 mm. (very late sign)! The PAT helps you to decide whether to give oxygen, whether to also give fluids, whether inotropes are needed and whether you need to call for help to intubate, severity and manage appropriately.

Table 1: Management of stridor based on etiology and severity of hypoxia.

Severity	ALTB: Prodrome, Brassy cough, hoarse voice 6 months–2 years	Epiglottis fever, toxic, drooling, dysphagia, hot potato voice 2–7 years	Retropharyngeal abscess: Fever, drooling, neck stiffness, torticollis < 5 years	FB: Playing with small objects, choking 6 months–5 years	Angioedema: Allergen
Stridor with no hypoxia	Steroids	Antibiotics ENT call over Shift to OT	Antibiotics ENT call over Shift to OT	ENT call over Shift to OT	Epinephrine Nebulization Epinephrine Deep IM Steroid Antihistamine
Stridcr with early hypoxia	Oxygen with CPAP Epinephrine Nebulization Steroid	Oxygen, Antibiotics ENT call over Shift to OT	Oxygen Antibiotics ENT call over Shift to OT	Oxygen ENT call over Shift to OT	Oxygen Epinephrine nebulization Epinephrine Deep IM Steroid Antihistamine

Contd...

Contd...

Stridor with severe hypoxia	Oxygen with CPAP NS Bolus : 10–20 ml/kg (if shock is identified) Epinephrine Nebulization Steroid	Oxygen with CPAP NS Bolus : 20–60 ml/kg ml/kg (if shock is identified) Dopamine infusion @ 10 mcg/kg/min if PE is noted during fluid therapy Antibiotics ENT call over Shift to OT	Oxygen with CPAP NS Bolus : 20–60 ml/kg (if shock is identified) Dopamine infusion @ 10 mcg/kg/min if PE is noted during fluid therapy Antibiotics ENT call over Shift to OT	Oxygen with CPAP NS Bolus : 5–10 ml/kg (if shock is identified)	Oxygen with CPAP NS Bolus : 20–200 ml/kg (if shock is identified) Epinephrine infusion
Stridor with late hypoxia	1. Bag valve mask ventilation followed by intubation and ventilation 2. Chest compression 15: 2 3. NS 10–20 ml/kg (bolus) 4. Epinephrine infusion 5. ENT call over for intubation in the ED (Anticipate difficult airway)				

KEY POINTS

1. Avoid separating mother and child.
2. Permit child to sit in a position of comfort.
3. Provide oxygen in a nonthreatening manner.
4. Determining anatomic level of obstruction enables appropriate management.
5. Assessment of severity helps to decide whether the child needs respiratory support in the ED or can wait to be shifted to the OT for definitive care.
6. Relying on pulse oximetry to determine severity of hypoxia can delay treatment.

Protocol 4.1: PEMC approach: Management of stridor in the emergency department

- Maintain child in position of comfort
- Avoid separation from mother
- Provide O_2 in non-threatening manner
- Laryngoscopic evaluation in an alert child with stridor is potentially lethal and can precipitate cardiac arrest

STRIDOR

Alert
Tone: N
Posture: N
Eyes: MP
EOM: N

Stable, obstructed
RR: N
WOB: N

HR: N
Perfusion: N
Color: N
BP: N
SaO_2: 100%

STRIDOR RESPIRATORY DISTRESS

Hyperalert
Tone: N
Posture: N

Stable, obstructed
RR: ↑
WOB: ↑

Tachycardia
Perfusion: N
Color: N
BP: N
SaO_2: 100%

STRIDOR RESPIRATORY FAILURE

Pain responsive/ unresponsive
Tone/posture: Abn
Abn eye position and movements
PERL

Unstable, obstructed
RR: ↑↓
WOB: ↑↓

HR: ↑↓
Shock
Color: Abn
BP: N
SaO_2: < 92%

NEUROGENIC STRIDOR

Unresponsive posturing
Unequal pupils
Abnormal eye position and movements
DEM: ±

Unstable obstructed apnea

Relative bradycardia
Perfusion: N/abn
Color: N/abn
BP: N↑
SaO_2: ≤100%

MANAGEMENT BASED ON ETIOLOGY

Etiology	Age	Fever	Cough	Voice	Stridor	Dysphagia	Others	Stridor	Stridor respiratory distress	Stridor respiratory failure	Neurogenic stridor
ALTB	3 m–5 y	±	Brassy	Hoarse	Harsh	–	–	Oral prednisolone 2 mg/kg stat or nebulized budesonide 2–4 mg/4 mL NS	Epinephrine nebulization 0.5 mg/kg up to maximum 5 mg (1:1,000) Inj. Dexamethasone 0.6 mg/kg IV/IM stat	Bag valve mask ventilation	Open airway
Epiglottitis	2 y–7 y	+++	Ineffective	Hot potato	Soft	+	Drooling of saliva	Rapid shift to E-OT accompanied by airway expert Avoid X-ray in ED Avoid laryngoscopic evaluation (even if ordered by ENT physician)	Rapid shift to E-OT accompanied by airway expert Avoid X-ray in ER	Shock correctoin Call for ENT/anesthetic help	Early intubation using **RSI** using ICP precautions for controlled ventilation Shock correction
RP abscess	< 5 y	+++	Ineffective	Muffled	Soft	+	Drooling of saliva, neck stiffness, torticollis	Rapid shift to E-OT accompanied by airway expert Avoid X-ray in ER Avoid laryngoscopic evaluation (even if ordered by ENT physician)	Rapid shift to E-OT accompanied by airway expert Avoid X-ray in ER	Plan to shift to OR **Avoid paralytic agents**	Evaluate for cause
FB aspiration	6 m–2 y	–	Sudden choking	Normal	Varies depending on site of obstruction	±	–	Plan shift to E-OT	Plan shift to E-OT		
Angioedema allergen +	Any	–	Dry staccato	Hoarse	Varies	±	Swelling of lips, tongue, mucus membrane, face	1. 100% O_2 through NRM 2. Early intubation by airway expert 3. Shock correction 4. Inj. Epinephrine 0.1 mg/kg IM (1:1,000) 5. Inj. Hydrocortisone 5 mg/kg IV 6. Inj. Diphenhydramine 1–2 mg/kg maximum 50 mg over 5–10 min IV 7. Inj. Ranitidine 1 mg/kg up to 50 mg IV 8. Salbutamol nebulization			

5
CHAPTER

Breathing

Chapter Outline

- How to recognize the cause for respiratory distress?
- How to recognize severity of hypoxia based on mother's history, rapid cardiopulmonary cerebral assessment and PAT?
- How to resuscitate based on etiology and severity of hypoxia?

INTRODUCTION

The commonest well known causes of respiratory distress in children are bronchiolitis, asthma, pneumonia.

The less well known but far more common cause of respiratory distress in shocked children is pulmonary edema.

Bronchiolitis

Inflammation of the bronchiolar mucosa occurs due to respiratory syncytial virus (RSV).

- An apparently trivial infection, the RSV infection causes mild fever, runny nose and a dry cough.

In infants from 6 months to 2 years of age the inflammation is not confined to the nasal mucosa. It spreads to the bronchiolar mucosa. These passages are tiny in this age group and tend to get blocked, resulting in rapid breathing with intercostal and subcostal recessions, feeding difficulty and wheeze on auscultation.

Asthma

This common cause of episodic respiratory distress affects healthy children beyond the age of 2 years.

Episodic respiratory distress in children less than 2 years is usually due to recurrent aspiration.

Asthma is an airway disease that can be classified as a partially reversible obstruction to air flow, with hypertrophy of the mucous glands, airway thickening due to inflammation, and bronchoconstriction, due to the tightening of the surrounding

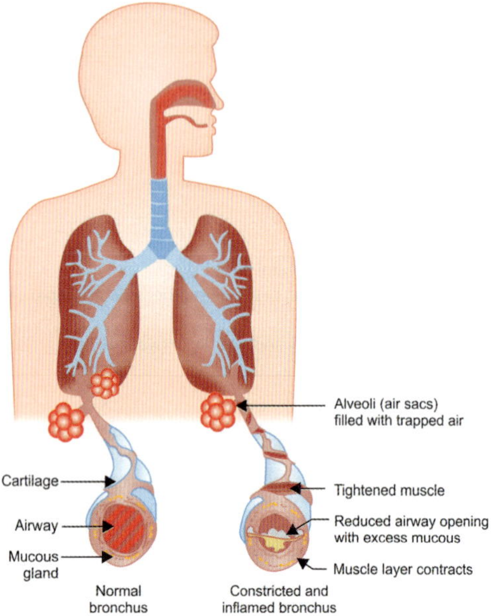

Figure 1: Pathophysiology of asthma: Bronchospasm, mucosal edema, increased secretion from the goblet cells and inflammation are characteristic features of asthma

smooth muscle. Bronchial inflammation also causes narrowing due to mucosal edema caused in response viral triggers (Figure 1).

Pneumonia

Pneumonia is an inflammatory condition of the lung, primarily affecting the alveoli.

Pneumonia, remains one of the commonest cause for acute onset of respiratory distress in the febrile child. Recognition and management of hypoxia, shock, cardiac dysfunction due to severe sepsis and appropriate antibiotics, can help reduce mortality.

It is commonly caused by viruses or bacteria (Figure 2).

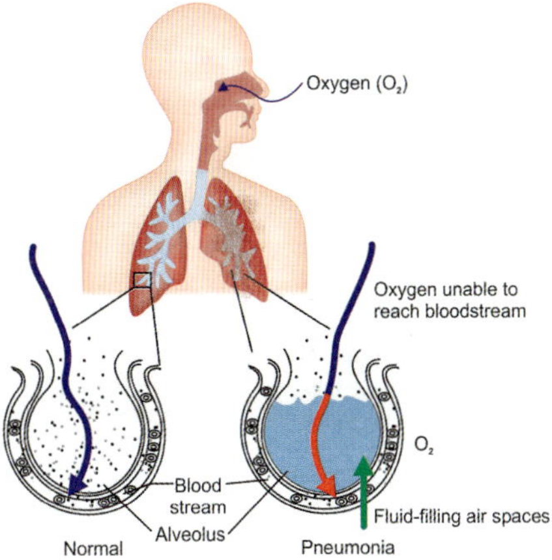

Figure 2: Pathophysiology of pneumonia

PULMONARY EDEMA

Cardiogenic Pulmonary Edema

Pulmonary edema is caused by rapid accumulation of fluid within the lung's interstitial and/or alveolar spaces. It results from the elevated cardiac-filling pressures.

Noncardiogenic Pulmonary Edema

The alveolar fluid accumulation is due to the movement of excess fluid into the alveoli due to leaky pulmonary capillaries (Figure 3).

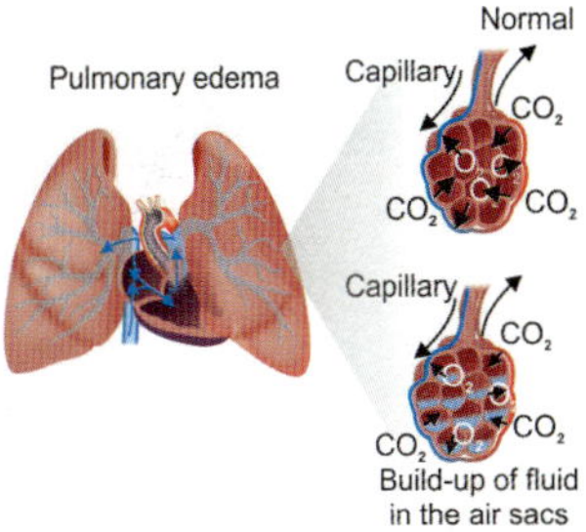

Figure 3: Pathophysiology of pulmonary edema: Pulmonary edema occurs due to accumulation of alveolar fluid

Approach to the child presenting with respiratory distress:

- Seat the child in his mom's lap. Avoid separating the child and his mom.
- Instruct mom to hold the oxygen mask. Care is taken to reduce anxiety (Avoid triggering crying).
- Gently, tie the age appropriate BP cuff.
- While, tying the cuff, ask targeted history for duration, pattern, etiology, comorbid conditions, medications and prehospital care.
- Whilst asking history, concurrently observe for vocalization (airway stability), retractions, pattern of respiration (abdominal or thoracic).
- Listen for stridor and grunt. Make note of the tone and posture. If flopping on his mom with closed eyes, presume "pain responsive". If , sitting up with eyes open, find out whether, as usual or not or less than alert. If mom reports not as usual, consider "responsive to voice".

Some findings need counting. Respiratory rate and heart rate (while counting, note whether heart sounds are note whether muffled or gallop). Compare pulses, assess core-peripheral temperature gap, color, CRT and liver span. Examine eyes for position and movements. Do not forget looking for pupillary response to light.

Fit your findings into the PAT. This will help to resuscitate appropriately (Figures 4A to D).

Respiratory distress without hypoxia

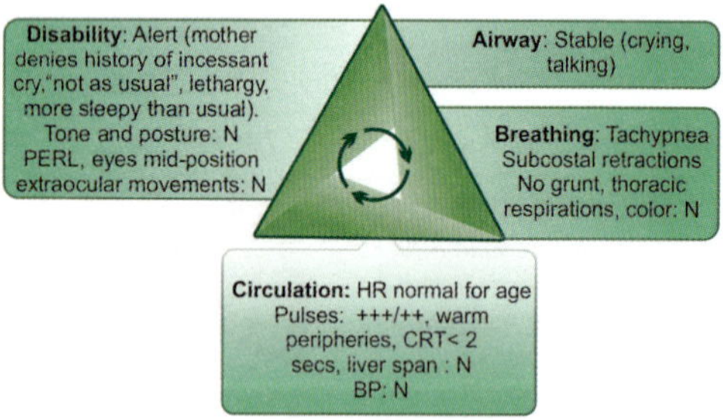

Figure 4A: Physiological status:
A: Stable (crying or talking); **B:** Respiratory distress; **C:** No tachycardia, no shock, BP normal for age, liver span normal for age; **D:** Alert (As per mom's history)

Note: Tachycardia can be precipitated by stranger anxiety. Hence, examination should be performed on the mother's lap in a non-threatening manner.

Respiratory distress with early hypoxia

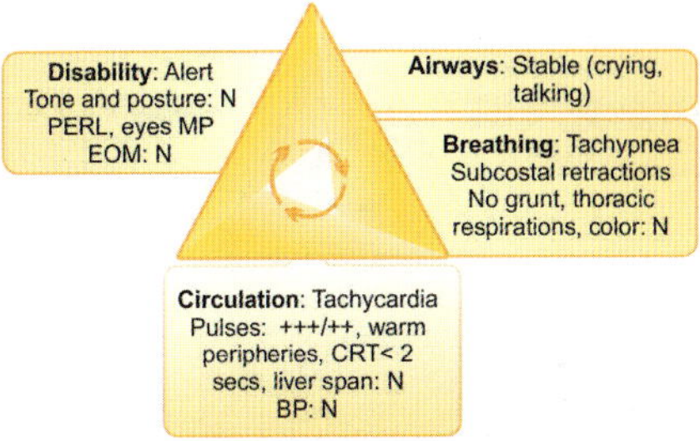

Figure 4B: Physiological status:
A: Stable (Cry or verbalizing); **B:** Respiratory distress; **C:** Tachycardia, no shock, liver span normal, BP normal; **D:** Alert

Respiratory distress with severe hypoxia

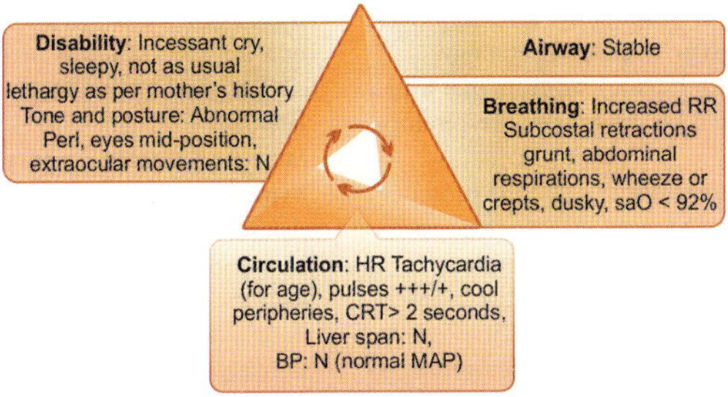

Figure 4C: Physiological status:
A: Stable with position; **B:** Impending respiratory failure; **C:** Tachycardia, shock, Liver span normal for age, BP Normal for age; **D:** ALC

Respiratory distress with late hypoxia (Respiratory failure)

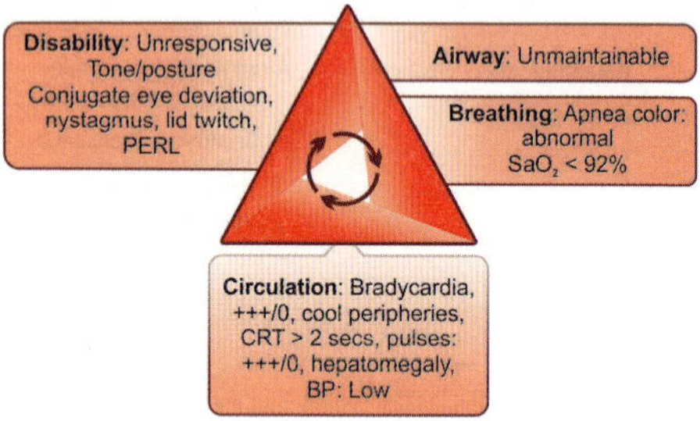

Figure 4D: Physiological status:
A: Unstable; **B:** Apnea; **C:** Bradycardia, hypotensive cardiogenic shock; **D:** ALOC, with Non-convulsive status epilepticus

Avoid rushing for a X-ray as the first intervention when a child presents with respiratory distress or respiratory failure.

Step 1: Targeted history to identify etiology

- Duration of respiratory distress offers many clues to the possible etiology.
- Hours (hyper acute) suggests that aspiration could be the cause of respiratory distress.
- Days (acute) indicates that the presence of an infective lung disease, e.g. pneumonia, empyema, bronchiolits, etc.
- Respiratory distress in months or since birth (chronic) implies that the possible etiology is cardiac or less commonly a chronic lung disease.
- Episodic breathlessness with symptom free periods, points towards asthma. Rarely, recurrent aspiration syndromes can present with episodic respiratory distress. Unlike asthmatic children, the latter is often associated with failure to thrive or developmental delay.
- Acute first episode of respiratory distress, associated with history of fever and non-lung foci of sepsis suggests the possibility of acute cardiogenic pulmonary edema.
- **Step 2: Targeted history to identify hypoxia or shock**
- Ask for history of altered mental status in any child presenting with respiratory distress. The mother is best judge. If she denies fall in mental status, the child is unlikely to have respiratory failure.
- Hypoxic or shocked kids can often talk or take feeds, therein misleading. His-tory of "not as usual", lethargy, sleepier than usual are more sensitive questions.

Step 3: Targeted history of fever suggests infective causes for respiratory distress
Example: Pneumonia, Bronchiolitis
Step 4: Cardiopulmonary cerebral assessment should be focused on recognizing:

Whether Respiratory Distress or Respiratory Failure

Classification of severity on arrival helps to establish urgency of treatment. Initiate bag valve mask ventilation if "BRADYNEIC". Further assessment, should be continued by the next responder.

Shock or Not

- It is not uncommon for shock to co-exist in hypoxic children. Early and energetic fluid shock resuscitation mandatory for early resolution of hypoxia.
- Respiratory distress and shock viz. cardiogenic shock may mimic asthma or bronchiolitis!
- When respiratory distress and shock is noted in children presenting with "non-lung etiologies" such as scorpion sting, septic foci, acute diarrhea, submersion injury, hypoxic ischemic encephalopathies, etc. suspect the presence of pulmonary edema due to cardiac dysfunction or acute lung injury.

Cardiogenic Shock or Not

- Examination of the liver span in a child with respiratory distress often provides valuable information on cardiac function. Since a pushed down liver could erroneously suggest hepatomegaly, emphasis is laid in assessment of the span. The upper border is percussed and marked. The lower border is palpated and a line is drawn parallel to the right costal margin. The span is measured in the mid-clavicular line. Assessment of the liver span during the cardiopulmonary assessment, helps to find out whether respiratory distress is due to respiratory or cardiac causes.
- Chronic respiratory distress associated with increased liver span, points towards a structural heart disease with cardiac failure.
- Acute respiratory distress, with increased liver span could occur due to cardiac failure or cardiogenic shock secondary to myocarditis or severe sepsis.

Subtle Status Epilepticus or not due to Severe Cerebral Hypoxia and Hypo-Perfusion

- Nystagmus, conjugate deviation or eye lid twitch or a combination of signs signal severe hypoxia in young children and infants. (Avoid treating with anticonvulsants).

> *Increased respiratory rates without increased work of breathing (quiet tachypnea), point towards a noncardiorespiratory cause of abnormal breathing patterns such as acidosis secondary to DKA, hypovolemic shock, etc.*

Comatose children present with altered breathing patterns secondary to neurogenic etiologies.

Treatment is focused on correction of hypoxia and shock concurrently with etiology (Table 1).

Table 1: Planning interventions based on etiology and severity of hyCpoxia for children presenting with respiratory distress

Severity	Bronchiolitis	Asthma	Pneumonia	Pulmonary edema
Respiratory distress with no hypoxia	Hydration	Salbutamol using MDI with spacer Steroid	Antibiotics	Anti-failure treatment
Respiratory distress with early hypoxia	Oxygen with CPAP 3% NS nebulization	Salbutamol 2.5 mg nebulization Oral steroid	Oxygen Antibiotics	Oxygen with CPAP
Respiratory distress with severe hypoxia	Oxygen with CPAP NS Bolus: 10–20 ml/kg (if shock is identified)	Oxygen with CPAP NS Bolus: 10–20 ml/kg (if shock is identified) Neb 2.5 mg Salbutamol+ Ipratropium 250–500 mcg Inj. Hydrocortisone	Oxygen with CPAP NS Bolus: 20–80 ml/kg (if shock is identified) Antibiotics	Oxygen with CPAP NS Bolus: 5–10 ml/kg (if shock is identified) Dopamine/dobutamine infusion @ 10 mcg/kg/minute when signs of pulmonary edema are noted during fluid resuscitation.
Respiratory failure with late hypoxia	Bag valve mask ventilation followed by intubation and ventilation Chest compression 15 : 2 NS 10–20 ml/kg (bolus) Epinephrine infusion Treatment of etiology			

Consider aspiration in children presenting with hyper-acute respiratory distress. Consider, bronchiolitis, in acute first episode of breathlessness, following prodrome. High grade fever, consider pneumonia.

- Oxygen with CPAP (if hypoxic as per PAT)
- Correct shock if noted
- Acute first episode breathlessness with wheeze in young healthy infants, presenting with low grade fever and prodrome is suggestive of bronchiolitis.
- Nebulization with hypertonic saline
- Epinephrine nebulization 0. 1 mL/kg (1:1000) in 4 mL of normal saline. Monitor ECG for cardiac arrhythmias, if hypertonic saline has not resolved respiratory distress.

First episode respiratory distress with or without hepatomegaly due to acute pulmonary edema.

- Oxygen through flow inflation ventilation device.
- Smaller aliquots of fluids
- Early inotrope infusion and early intubation may be needed.

Episodic breathlessness in healthy children more than 2 years of age is probably asthma.

Grade severity and implement as per asthma protocol guidelines (Table 2). How to prepare the nebulizer solution for a child presenting with asthma complicated by severe hypoxia (Figures 5 A to G).

Caution: Avoid treating all respiratory distress with wheeze as asthma. Acute cardiogenic or noncardiogenic pulmonary edema, bronchiolitis may also present with wheeze.

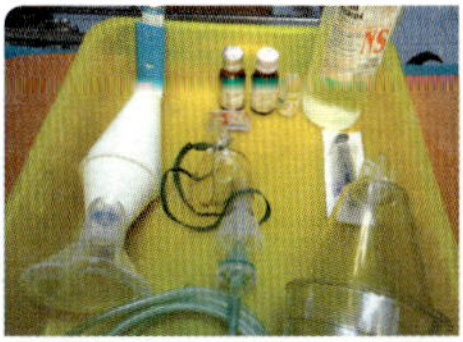

Figure 5A: Equipment and drugs needed for nebulization

1. a. Nebulizer chamber
   b. Spacer is used for children presenting with asthma without hypoxia (moderate asthma)
2. Nebulizer solutions:
   a. Salbutamol: 1 ml contains 2.5 mg
   b. Ipratropium Bromide: 1 ml contains 250 micrograms
3. Normal saline: 2-3 ml of NS is needed to ensure nebulization. (distilled water is not used since salbutamol does not dissolve in distilled water. Distilled water also irritates the airway)
4. Steroid
   a. T. Prednisolone: Full dose is taken stat.
   b. Injection Hydrocortisone: Indicated for hypoxic asthmatics, vomiting or when unable to swallow prednisolone.

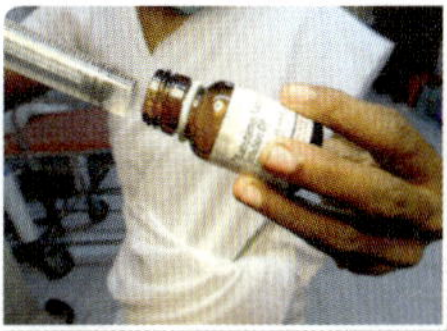

Figure 5B: Withdraw 2.5 mg (0.5 cc) salbutamol solution with a clean syringe. Note: 2.5 mg is used for all ages. The dose is based on minute ventilation and not weight.

Caution: Salbutamol nebulization can worsen hypoxia and can precipitate cardiac arrest in children presenting with non-asthmatic causes of respiratory distress. Remember that "All that wheezes is not asthma"

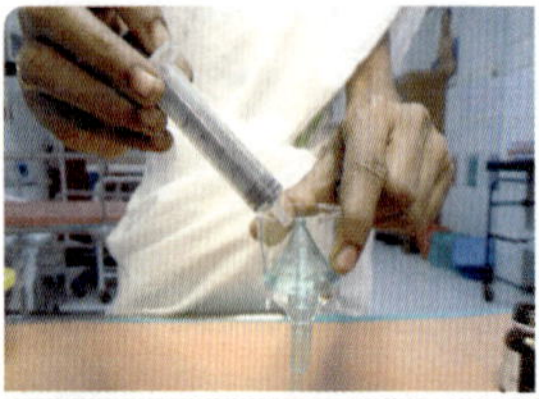

Figure 5C: Add the salbutamol in to the chamber.

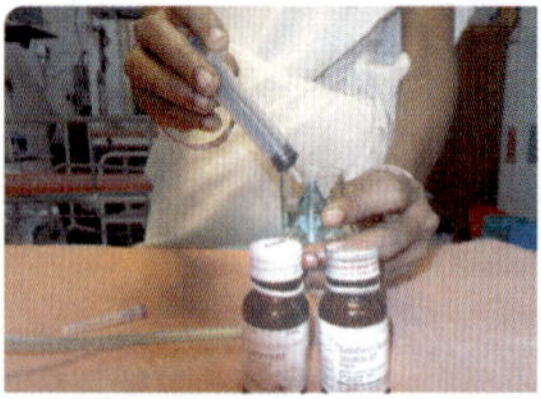

Figure 5E: Add Ipratropium bromide to the nebulizing chamber.

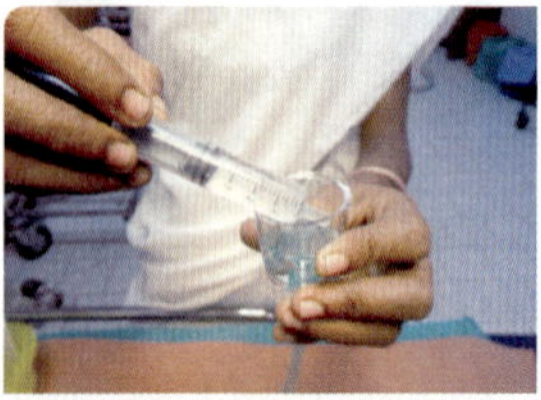

Figure 5G: Add NS to the nebulizing chamber

Figure 5A to G: How to load the nebulizing chamber with Salbutamol, Ipratropium Bromide and NS.

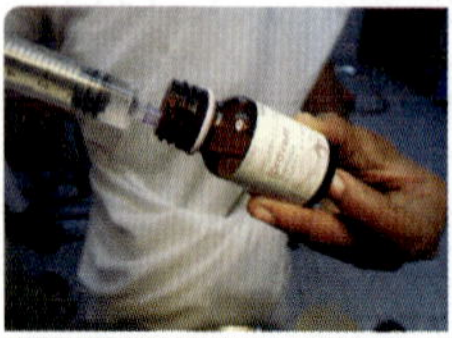

Figure 5D: Withdraw Ipravent (2 ml contains 500 mcg using an empty syringe. Ipratropium Bromide, is useful only in hypoxic asthmatics. It acts on the cholinernergic receptors that are only found in the larger airways.

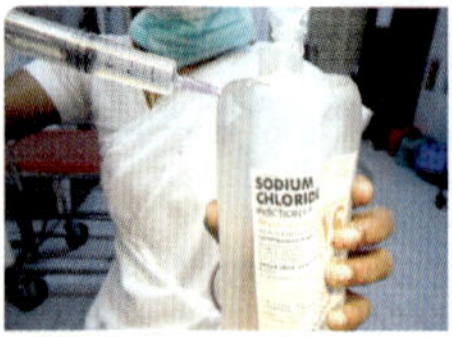

Figure 5F:

Caution during Nebulization:

1. Confirm, that the etiology of respiratory distress is asthma
2. Confirm, that the child is having hypoxia. (Use spacer for non-hypoxic asthma.
3. Always nebulize on the mother's lap (Mother is the best monitor if the mental status deteriorates during nebulization)
4. Connect the nebulizing chamber to the oxygen source to drive the bronchodilator drugs.
5. Perform the rapid cardiopulmonary cerebral assessment after each nebulization. Note if triangle shifts to green, nebulization can be withheld.
6. Keep the bag valve mask handy.
7. Connect pulse oximeter.
8. Steroids, should be given within 30 minutes of treatment for acute exacerbation.

Table 2: Drugs used for asthmatic exacerbation in the ED

	Drugs	Route	Dose	Side Effects	Remarks
1.	Salbutamol	Nebulized	2.5 mg in 4 ml normal saline.	Tremors, nausea, tachycardia Blood pressure instability, Cardiac arrhythmias Myocardial instability Beware: Salbutamol nebulization, worsens hypoxia, occasionally leading to cardiac arrest in very hypoxic children when given for nonasthmatic causes of respiratory distress	Hypokalemia occurs Prolongation QTc interval
2.	Ipratropium	Nebulized	250–500 ug Q4–6 hrly	Rarely mydriasis and blurred vision	Peak responses develop after 30–90 mins
3.	Hydrocortisone	IV	2–4 mg/kg Q6 hrly	Hypertension, hyperglycemia, mood disorders, gastritis	Always give H_2 blocker as prophylaxis for gastritis and to prevent perforation. Short course for 5–7 days. After the acute course is over, can be changed to oral
4.	Methylprednisolone	IV	0.5–1 mg/kg/dose Q6 hrly	Hypertension, hyperglycemia, mood disorders, gastritis	Always give H_2 blocker as prophylaxis for gastritis and to prevent perforation. Short course for 5–7 days. After the acute course is over, can be changed to oral
5.	Adrenaline	SC	0.1 ml/kg (1:10,000)	Tachycardia, hypertension	Administered in near fatal asthma
6.	Terbutaline	IV	Loading dose: 10 mg/kg over 10 mins Infusion: 0.1 mg/kg/min	Same as salbutamol but more pronounced	Subcutaneous doses can be tried before giving IV infusion. Adrenaline can be used alternatively

Contd...

Contd...

	Drugs	Route	Dose	Side Effects	Remarks
		SC	0.01 mg/kg dose for 3 doses Q20 min		
7.	Aminophylline	IV	Loading dose: 1.25 mg/kg/dose Over 20 mins < 6 months: 0.5 mg/kg/hr 6 months to 1 year: 0.85–1 mg/kg/hr 1–9 yrs: 1 mg/kg/hr > 9 yrs: 0.75 mg/kg/hr	Nausea, vomiting, fever, dyskinesia, seizures and death	Extremely narrow therapeutic index. Hence, decrease dose in patients with hepatic and cardiovascular dysfunction.
8.	Magnesium sulfate	IV	25–50 mg/kg/dose over 20–30 mins	Hypotension, nausea, flushing arrhythmias, muscle weakness, areflexia and respiratory depression	No role for continuous infusion

KEY POINTS

1. Avoid separating mother and child during assessment of a child presenting with respiratory distress.
2. Teach mom to hold the oxygen mask in a non-threatening manner.
3. Focused history with emphasis on duration provides clues to the possible etiology.
4. History of altered level of consciousness helps recognize early signs of hypoxia in a child presenting with respiratory distress.
5. Rapid cardiopulmonary assessment, which incorporates assessment of liver span, helps to recognize whether respiratory distress is due to respiratory or cardiac causes.

Protocol 5.1: PEMC approach: Respiratory distress

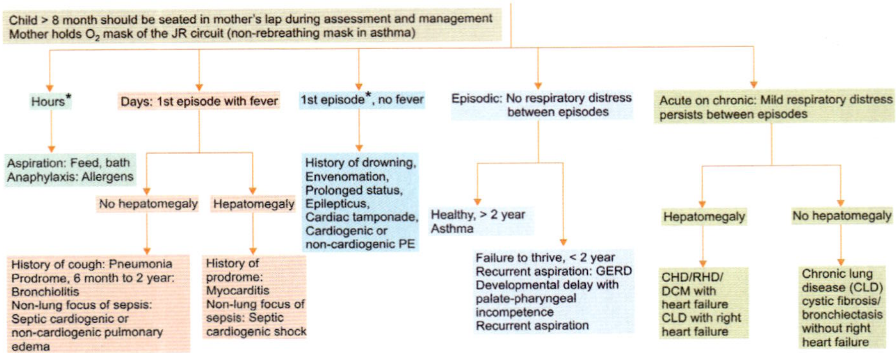

All that wheezes is not asthma, probe history to avoid potentially lethal complications of salbutamol nebulization in hypoxic children with respiratory distress

- Bronchospasm: Asthma (episodic), anaphylaxis
- Bronchiolar edema: Bronchiolitis (1st episode)
- Mucus plugs: Cystic fibrosis (acute on chronic)
- Interstitial/alveolar edema compressing bronchioles: Pulmonary edema

1. Chronic respiratory distress-congenital heart disease
2. Acute 1st episode respiratory distress with non-lung focus of sepsis: Septic cardiogenic shock
3. Pulmonary capillary leak: Acute lung injury occurs, can occur in serious illness of any etiology

Suprasternal and sternal retractions: Suspect upper airway obstruction,intercostal, subcostal retractions-consider lung pathology

Effortless tachypnea: DKA, metabolic acidosis (normal lung)

Infants < 2 month of age

- First episode, hyperacute/acute respiratory distress, consider CHD
- Recurrent episodes in < 2 year with FTT/ immunocompromise, consider recurrent pneumonia
- Acute respiratory distress with failure to thrive, consider CCF or CLD despite negative history
- Hepatomegaly with effortless tachypnea, consider intrinsic liver

Protocol 5.2: PEMC approach: Management of acute exacerbation of asthma

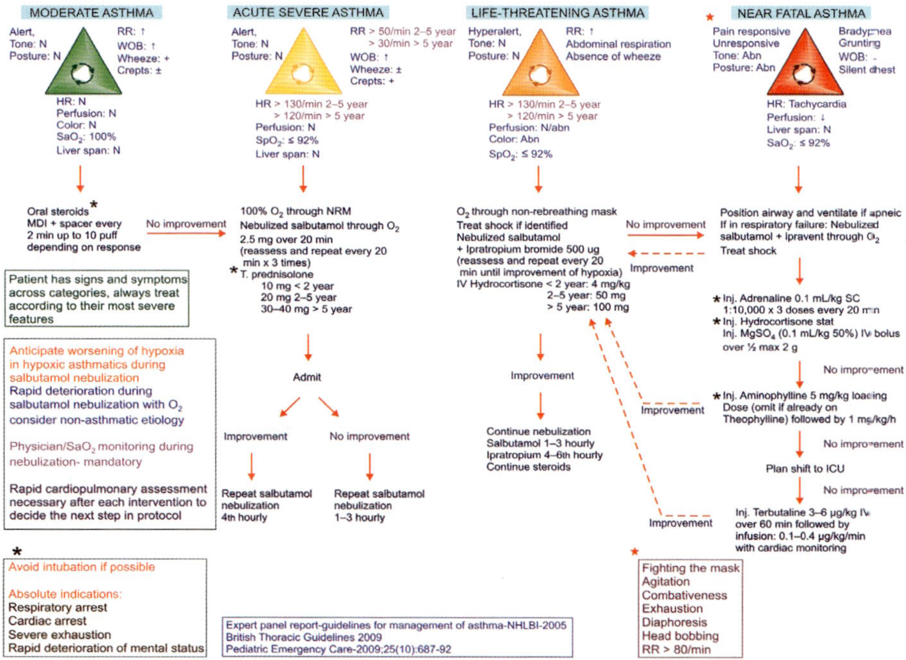

6 CHAPTER Circulation

Chapter Outline

- Hypovolemic shock
- Septic shock
- Dengue shock
- Anaphylactic shock
- Obstructive shock
- How to secure intra-osseous when IV access is not easily available?

HYPOVOLEMIC SHOCK

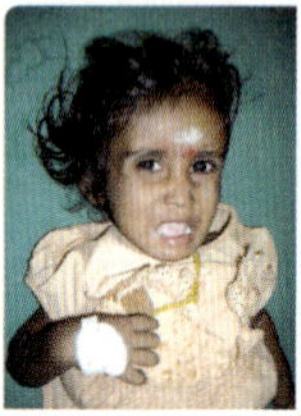

Sunken eyes due to severe dehydration. Note also the irritable look. Mother's history of incessant cry, followed by the rapid cardiopulmonary cerebral assessment helped identify shock.

PATHOPHYSIOLOGY

Acute diarrheal loss of fluids results in the following:

Features of Dehydration

- Sunken eyes
- Dry mucosa
- Sunken anterior fontanelle
- Thirst
- Loss of skin turgor

Loss of volume exceeding 25% of effective circulating volume leads to decreased cerebral perfusion and fall in the level of consciousness (incessant cry, sleepy, lethargic, not as usual)

Severe dehydration is attributed to loss of 10% circulating volume which is not sufficient to cause decreased cerebral perfusion.

Unfortunately, severe dehydration is often equated to shock.

- The approach described below uses the pediatric assessment triangle (PAT) to identify severity of illness in acute watery diarrhea (AWD) Figure 1.

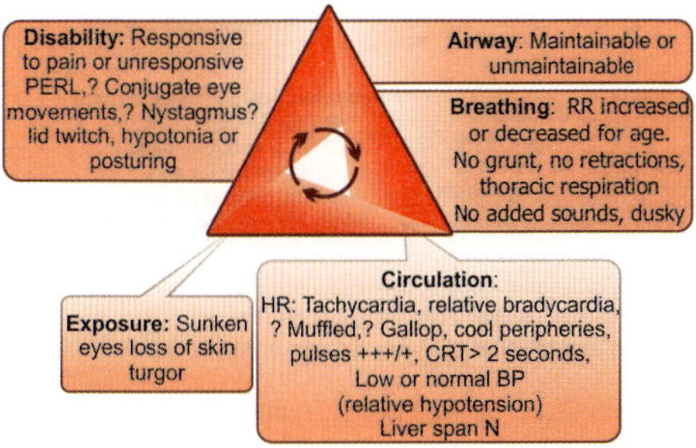

Figure 1: Hypotensive shock due to hypovolemia.

Physiological status: Airway stable or not stable/effortless tachypnea or bradypnea/hypotensive shock/altered mental status with or without nonconvulsive status epilepticus with severe dehydration.

Management

- Provide oxygen using the nonrebreathing mask.
- Secure 2 IV lines and infuse RL 20 mL/kg using pull push technique until BP normalizes for age.
- Check dextrostix and correct documented hypoglycemia.
- Repeat rapid cardiopulmonary cerebral assessment after every fluid bolus until BP normalizes.

Avoid antibiotics, since most diarrheal episodes are secondary to viral infections.

- If cholera is suspected (as in this child) oral doxycycline should be prescribed.
- If dysentery or less than 6 months of age or has systemic illness or has proven or suspicion of shigellosis, initiate the appropriate antimicrobial.

Severe Dehydration (Figure 2)

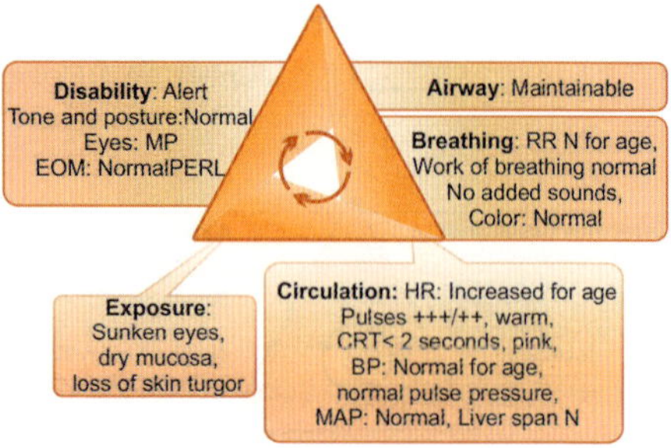

Figure 2: Airway stable/breathing normal/tachycardia, no shock/alert. Dehydration, as evidenced by sunken eyes and loss of skin turgor. Persistent tachycardia is an early sign of severe dehydration.

Management of Severe Dehydration Without Shock

- Discontinue oxygen therapy.
- *Children > 1 year:* 30 mL/kg (within 30 minutes); then 70 mL/kg in the next 2 hours.
- *Children < 1 year:* 30 mL/kg in the 1st hour; then 70 mL/kg in the next 5 hours.

Diarrhea with some Dehydration (Figure 3)

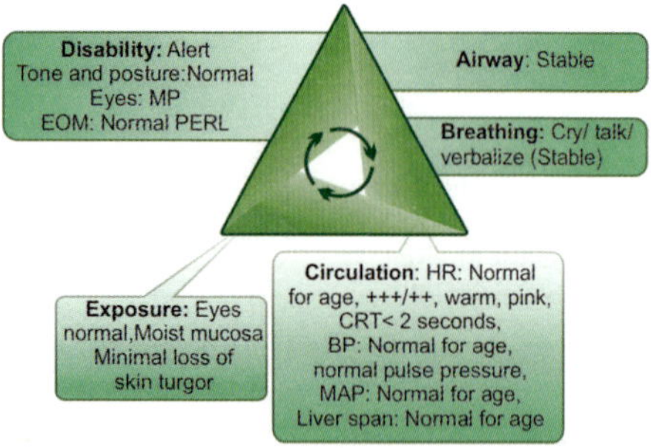

Figure 3: Airway: Stable, breathing: Normal, Circulation: HR normal, no shock, BP: Normal, Pulse pressure normal, MAP normal, No hepatomegaly, Disability: Nil, Some dehydration (3–5% loss of fluids).

Management of Diarrhea with some Dehydration

- Advise ORS 75 mL/kg for 4 hours and review.
- ORS ad lib in the older child.

Diarrhea with no Dehydration (< 3% Loss of Fluids)

Acute diarrhea is defined by the World Health Organization (WHO) as the passage of three or more loose or liquid stools per day, for three or more days and for less than 14 days.

Management

- ORS—10 mL/kg for every loose stool.

KEY POINTS

1. Repeat cardiopulmonary cerebral assessment after every fluid order. Recurrence of diarrheal episodes and vomiting can alter the physiological status.
2. Attempt to shift the pediatric assessment triangle from the shock triangle to the normal triangle.
3. Inotropes and intubation are rarely needed in the management of uncomplicated hypovolemic shock.

Protocol 6.1: PEMC approach: Recognition of the severity of dehydration and presence of septic shock in children presenting with diarrhea

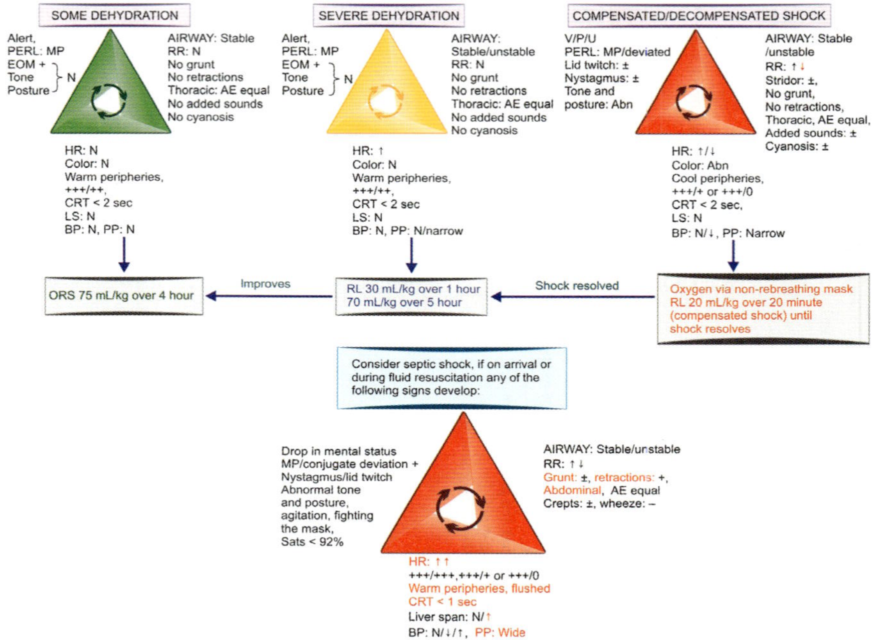

SEPTIC SHOCK

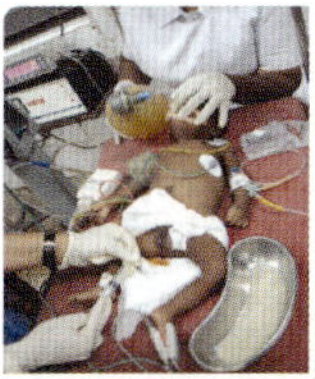

Source control. Draining abscess during resuscitation of septic shock is crucial for successful outcomes.

PATHOPHYSIOLOGY

In some children, infection triggers a dysregulated host response leading to life-threatening organ dysfunction.

- **Dysregulated host response:** This means that the host releases an excessive quantity of inflammatory mediators in response to microbial invasion.
- **Life-threatening organ dysfunction:** The inflammatory mediators damage the endothelial cells lining both the systemic and pulmonary circulation. The resultant vasodilation and capillary leak in the systemic circulation causes shock. The leak in the pulmonary circulation causes pulmonary edema in the lungs (Figure 4).

Some of the interleukins (cytokines) also cause severe cardiac dysfunction leading to cardiogenic pulmonary edema.

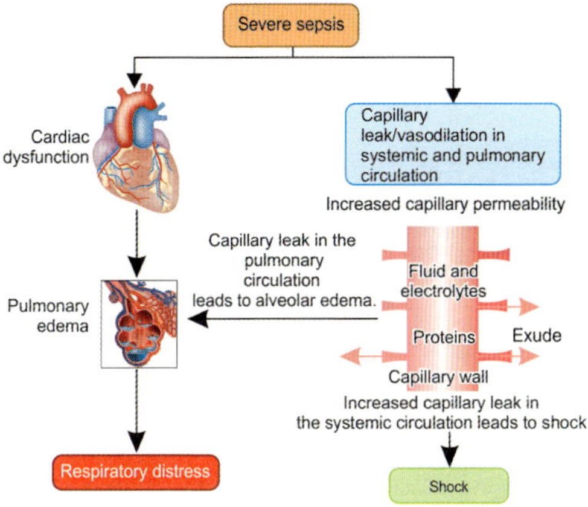

Figure 4: Pathophysiology of organ dysfunction in severe sepsis.

How do we recognize life-threatening organ dysfunction in children presenting with fever?

1. Triage question:
   Ask the mother whether her child with fever and focus (AWD, otitis, cellulitis, etc.) has incessant cry, is lethargic, more sleepy than usual or "not as usual"!

Fall in mental status in a child with fever or diarrhea suggests cerebral hypoperfusion or shock.

How do we recognize whether a child with fever and focus of infection has early pulmonary edema due to severe sepsis?

2. Triage question:
   Find out whether the child has developed breathlessness (not episodic or since birth)

History of *breathlessness,* in children, presenting with altered mental status and shock, helps to recognize pulmonary edema secondary to acute lung injury or cardiac dysfunction (Figure 5).

The early recognition of sepsis with life-threatening organ dysfunction by interns has been possible by simple clinical tools.

- Probing for history of altered mental status and breathlessness in every child who presents with fever and foci.
- Performance of the rapid cardio-pulmonary cerebral assessment
- Using the PAT to derive vasodilatory cardiogenic shock with or without non-convulsive status epilepticus.

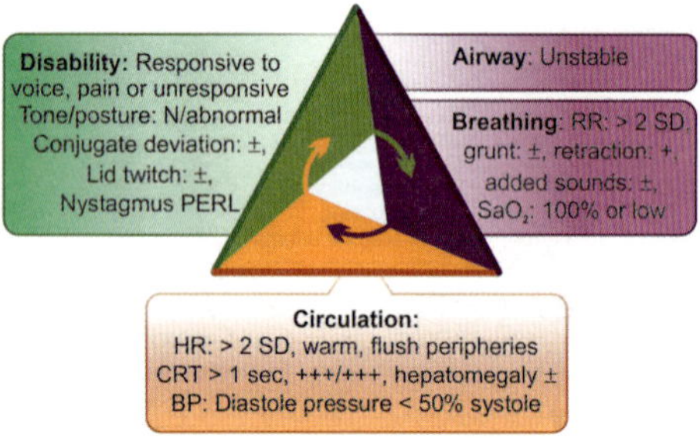

Figure 5: Respiratory distress/failure with vasodilatory cardiogenic shock with our without non-convulsive status epilepticus.

Management of Septic Shock with Pulmonary Edema

Fluids are the cornerstone of shock resuscitation. But pulmonary edema (PE) is an inherent complication of severe sepsis.

How do we resuscitate shock despite the risk of pulmonary edema?

- Oxygen is provided using a CPAP device (Flow inflating ventilation device) for the spontaneously breathing child (Figure 6).

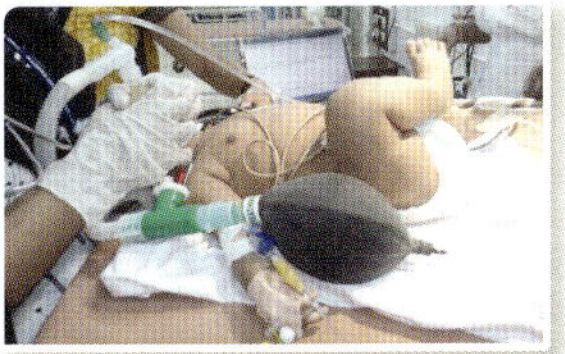

Figure 6: Oxygen is being provided via the Jackson-Rees circuit.

- If apneic, initiate bag valve mask ventilation (Figure 7).

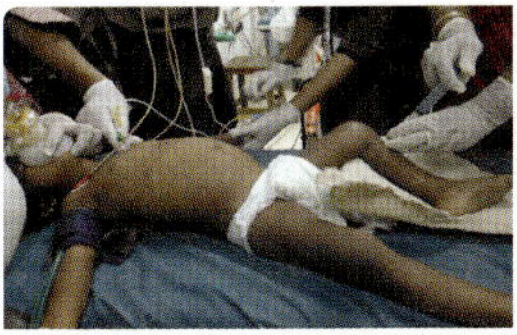

Figure 7: Bag valve mask ventilation in progress. Concurrently, fluids being bolused via the intraosseous route. A needle thoracocentesis has been performed for pneumothorax.

- IV or IO access is secured. Two intravenous access are necessary in the management of shock.
- Nonglucose containing isotonic fluids such as normal saline (NS) or Ringer's lactate—RL) are the fluids of choice.
- Dose: 20 mL/kg boluses over 20 minutes, if the child is normotensive for age (by gravity).
- If the child has respiratory distress and normotensive shock, the bolus is smaller 5–10 mL/kg over 5–10 minutes (by gravity).
- Pull push technique is used only, if hypotension is documented (age appropriate cuffs should be used to assess BP).
- If BP becomes normotensive, further boluses are administered by gravity.
- Rapid cardiopulmonary cerebral assessment is repeated after each bolus.

Fluid boluses are continued until therapeutic goals of shock and pulmonary edema are resolved (Figure 8).
Glucose/normal saline or dextrose only (5% or 10%) is not recommended for shock correction.

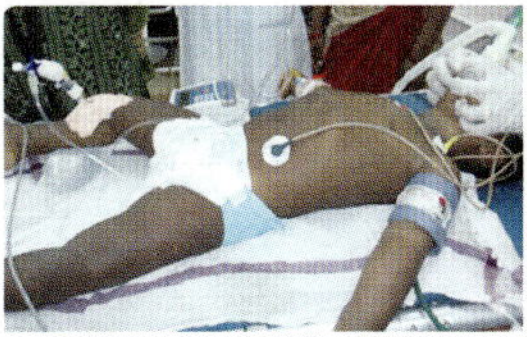

Figure 8: The airway is being positioned. Oxygen is being administered using a JR circuit. An intraosseous line has been secured. Later, IV access has also been secured. The IO line is dedicated for inotrope infusion.

- Documented hypoglycemia is corrected with 2 mL/kg of 25% dextrose. Glucose containing maintenance fluids are initiated throughout resuscitation.
- Blood is collected for CBC, smear for malaria, cultures, MSAT, scrub. urine and other body fluids may be collected and sent for cultures. Blood is also sent for RFT, LFT, electrolytes, grouping and cross-matching.

Antibiotics

- Ceftriaxone is administered at 100 mg/kg in children more than 3 months of age.
- Cefotaxime (200 mg/kg) with Ampicillin (200 mg/kg) is administered in infants less than 3 months of age.
- Azithromycin 10 mg/kg, if fever for more than 5 days with or without eschar.
- Artesunate 2.4 mg/kg, if malaria is proven.

During fluid therapy, if signs of pulmonary edema are unmasked, interrupt fluids, initiate an inotrope, and refer to higher center (Figure 9 and Table 1).

Continue Oxygen via CPAP, fluids and inotrope until shock and pulmonary edema are resolved (Figure 10).

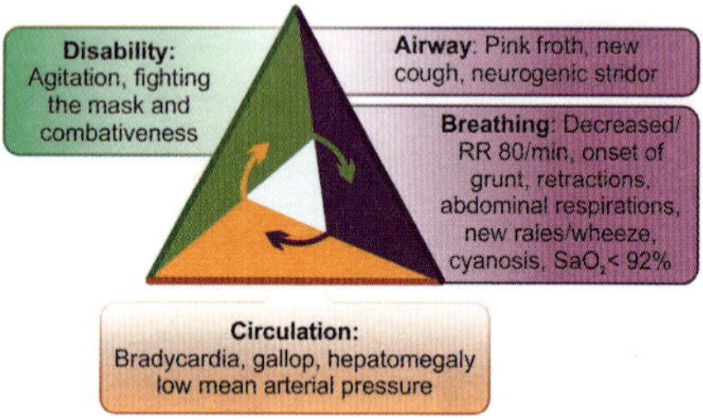

Figure 9: When to start inotropes during fluid therapy.

Caution: These are signs of pulmonary edema (heart failure). If these signs are ignored, and fluid is continued without application of inotropes or CPAP/ET, cardiac arrest can supervene.

Table 1: Preparation of inotropes.

Preparation of vasoactive agents Name of drug	When to start	Rule of 6 Add to 100 mL	Rule of 3 Add to 50 mL	If rate of administration is 10 mL/hour
Epinephrine	Hypotensive shock Caution: 1. Use correct sized cuff to document BP 2. Check age related BP values 3. The other parts of the pediatric triangle should be grossly abnormal	0.6 mg × Body weight	0.3 mg × Body weight	0.05 to 1 µg/kg/minute
Norepinephrine	Dopamine refractory vasodilatory shock	0.6 mg × Body weight	0.3 mg × Body weight	0.3 to 1 µg/kg/minute
Dopamine	Shock with normal systole pressure with vasodilation (diastole lower than 50% of systole) Caution: Dopamine (only after fluid bolus) (Dopamine cannot be initiated without establishing euvolemia (fluid resuscitation) Dopamine is indicated only when inotrope triggers or signs of pulmonary edema manifest during fluid resuscitation for correction of shock (Figure 9).	6 mg × Body weight	3 mg × Body weight	10 µg/kg/minute
Dobutamine	High systolic pressure with narrow pulse pressure shock 1. Dobutamine is initiated only after fluid resuscitation. 2. When inotrope triggers or signs of pulmonary edema manifest* (Figure 9).	6 mg × Body weight	3 mg × Body weight	10 µg/kg/minute

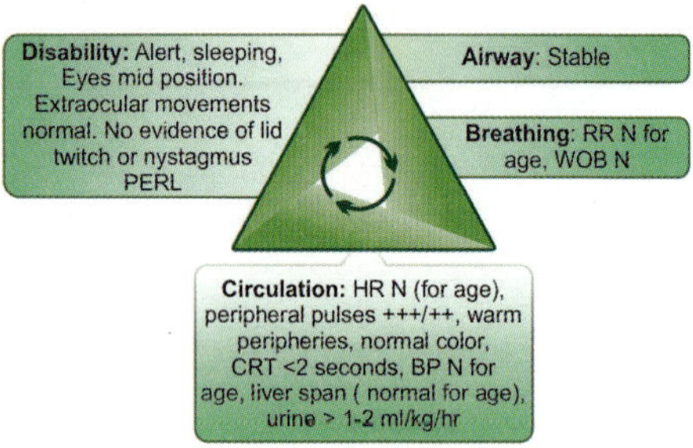

Figure 10: CPAP, fluids and inotropes should be administered until therapeutic goals of shock and pulmonary edema are resolved.

Recognition and Management of Septic Shock (Figure 11)

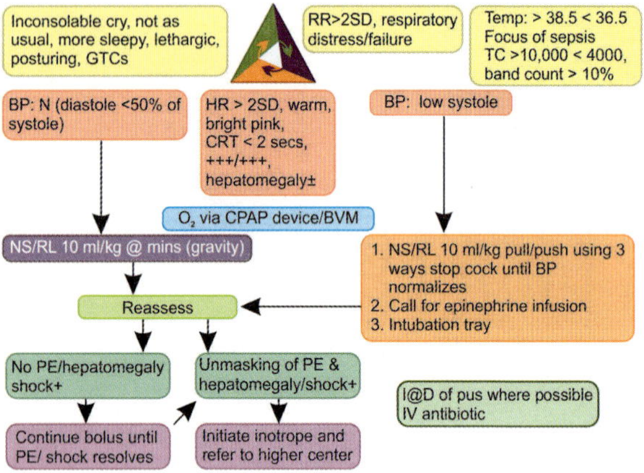

Figure 11: Protocol for initial management of septic shock.

KEY POINTS

1. Recognize septic shock by looking for evidence of decreased mental status and peripheral perfusion in any ill-looking child with fever.
2. Altered level of consciousness in a febrile child could be due to septic shock. Correction of the hypoxia and shock often improves mental status in the ED.
3. Resuscitation should be continued till all therapeutic goals of shock and pulmonary edema are resolved.

Protocol 6.2: PEMC approach: Early recognition of septic shock in the out patient department

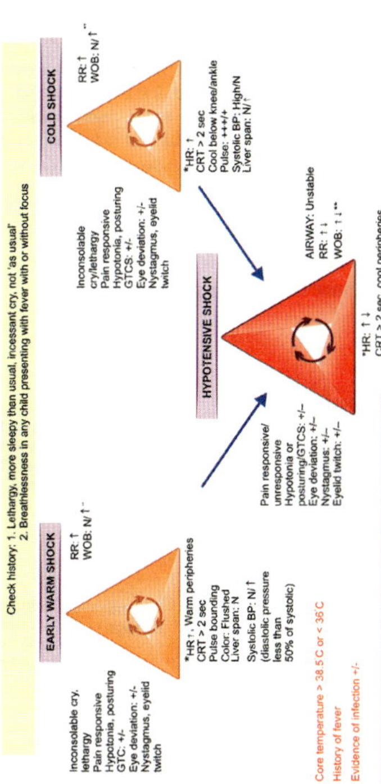

- Core temperature > 38.5°C or < 36°C
- History of fever
- Evidence of infection +/-

Age	*Heart rate		**Respiratory rate	Systolic BP
< 1 year	> 180	< 100	> 60 or requiring respiratory support	< 70 mm Hg
2–5 year	> 140	< 90	> 50 or requiring respiratory support	< 70 + age x 2
6–12 year	> 130		> 18 or requiring respiratory support	< 70 + age x 2 up to 10 year < 90 beyond 10 year

Age related vital signs required to recognize SIRS: International Sepsis Forum- 2005

*Respiratory distress with shock in a hypo- or hyperthermic child with or without focus of sepsis consider:

1. Pneumonia with shock.
2. Pulmonary edema with shock.
3. If respiratory distress/failure occurs or worsens during fluid resuscitation, consider pulmonary edema due to severe sepsis.

Dengue Shock

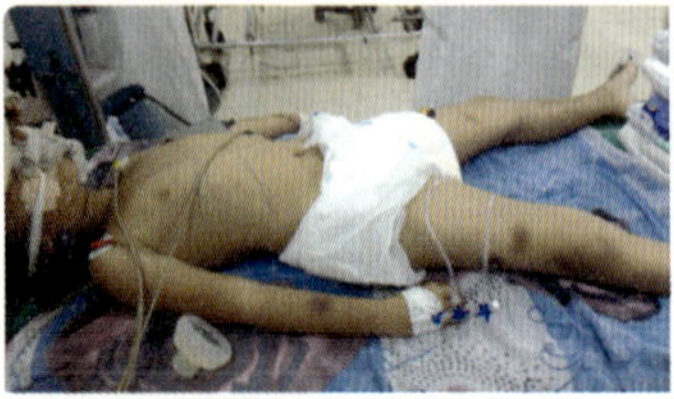

PATHOPHYSIOLOGY

Cytokines released in response to Dengue virus, cause vascular permeability and platelet dysfunction. The resultant loss of intravascular fluids leads to shock. Platelet destruction and dysfunction predisposes to bleeding tendencies. During the critical phase (leaky phase), hematocrit rises and platelets fall resulting in thrombocytopenia. (Figure 12).

Although, attention is focused on thrombocytopenia, it is the monitoring of hematocrit, frequent rapid cardiopulmonary cerebral assessment and urine output, that helps in achieving successful outcomes.

Dengue might present in the febrile, critical (risk of shock) or in the recovery phase (Figure 13).

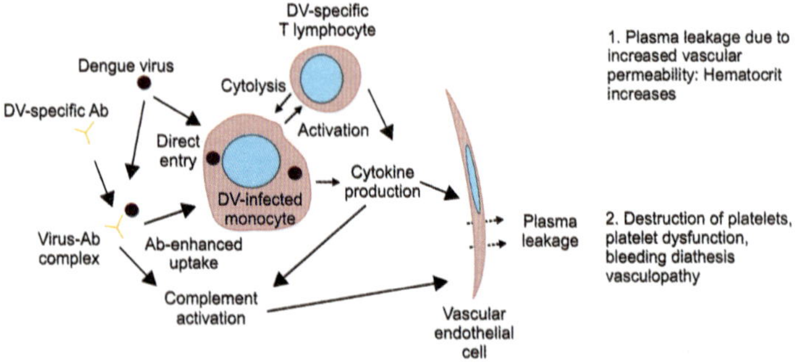

Figure 12: Pathophysiology of dengue.

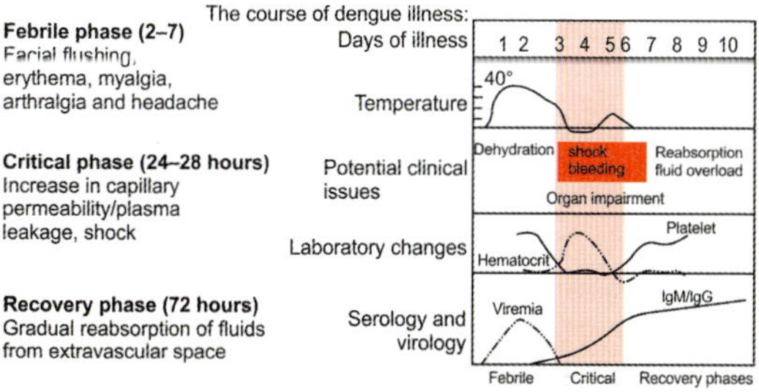

Figure 13: What are the three phases of dengue?

A FEBRILE EPISODE MAY BE DENGUE (WHO CRITERIA)

Fever and 2 of the following criteria:

- Nausea/vomiting
- Aches and pains
- Rash
- Tourniquet test positive
- Leucopenia with or without NS1 positivity (important when no signs of plasma leakage are identified).

Triage Questions

1. Mom denies history of child being more sleepy than usual, lethargy, inconsolable cry (infants). The child has been his usual self!
2. Denies history of breathlessness.

Hess test: The BP cuff is elevated mid-way between systole and diastole and held for 10 minutes. Development of at least 15 petechiae in a 5 cm² area is considered positive tourniquet test.

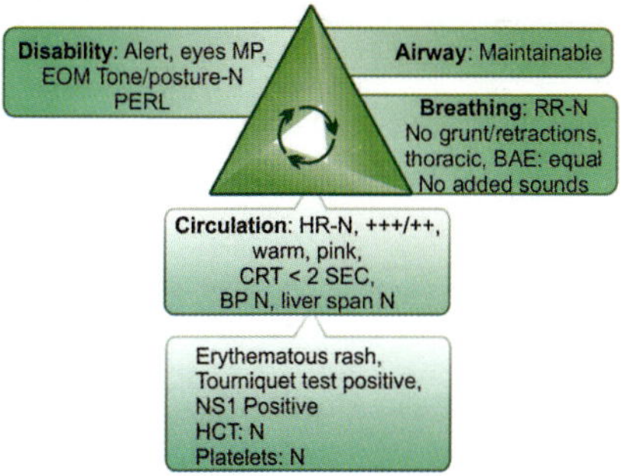

Figure 14: Probable dengue.

Management of Probable Dengue (Figure 14)

- Bed rest at home
- Instruct mom to maintain urine output chart (Table 2)
- Adequate fluid intake: ORS, fruit juice (Table 3)
- Paracetamol 10 mg/kg
- Teach them warning signs.

Table 2: Intake/output chart maintained by the mother.

Date	Time	What fluid	Input (mL)	Time	Output (mL)

Table 3: Daily requirement of ORS (recommended by the WHO) for fluid resuscitation of dengue.

Body weight in kg	ORS (ml/kg/day)
> 3–10	100
> 10–20	75
> 20–30	50–60
> 30–60	40–50

DENGUE WITH WARNING SIGNS (FIGURE 15)

- Abdominal pain or tenderness
- Persistent vomiting
- Fluid accumulation
- Mucosal bleed
- Liver enlargement > 2 cm

Laboratory Signs

- Increase in HCT (20% more than baseline) > 36%
- Rapid decrease in platelet count.

Triage History

1. Mom, denies history of fall in mental status or breathlessness.

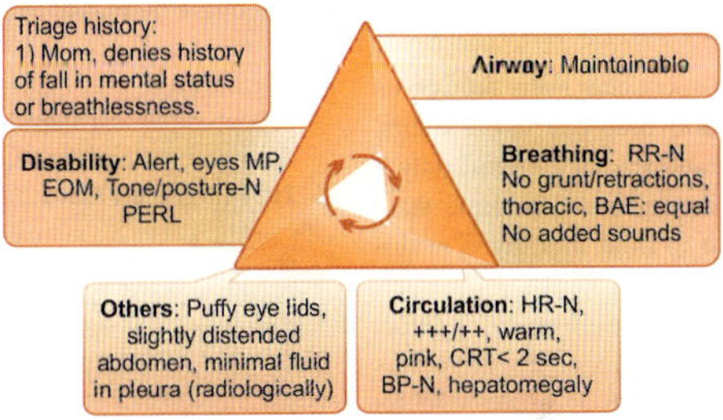

Figure 15: Dengue with warning signs (hemodynamically normal).

Management of Hemodynamically Stable Dengue with Warning Signs (Figure 15)

- Cardiopulmonary assessment is repeated every hour during the critical phase.
- Urine output should be monitored 4-6 hourly.
- HCT is repeated after fluid therapy, and 6-12 hourly thereafter.

If Hematocrit Remains the Same or Increases Minimally and Cardiopulmonary Assessment is Stable

- NS is continued at the rate of 2-3 ml/kg/hour for another 2-4 hours.
- Oral fluids are initiated once the child tolerates oral.
- Oral fluids/ORS are initiated once the child tolerates oral intake Table 2 and 3.

If HCT, increases rapidly and clinical deterioration occurs (Figure 16):

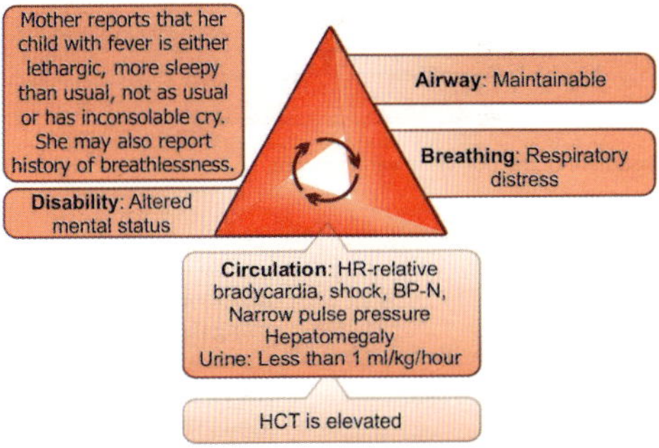

Figure 16: Dengue with warning signs and compensated shock.

- Ensure that urine output is > 0.5 mL/kg/ hour.
- Monitor hematocrit after every fluid bolus until stable and then every 4–6 hours.
- The interpretation is meaningful only if the corresponding hemodynamic state and response to fluid therapy is evaluated simultaneously.
- Random HCT in the absence of information about the hemodynamic status or response to fluids is unlikely to be useful.
- If shock is noted (Figure 16), initiate Oxygen via JR circuit
- Fluids are increased to 10 ml/kg over one hour.
- Further fluid administration is based on repeat rapid cardiopulmonary cerebral assessment and repeat evaluation of HCT (Figures 17 and 20).

Caution: Fluids are titrated to normal clinical goals of shock resolution and urine output of 0.5 ml/kg/hour. Total daily fluids should not exceed 1.5 times maintenance.

Ideal body weight is used for calculation of fluid infusion in obese children. Intravenous fluids are required only for 24–48 hours.

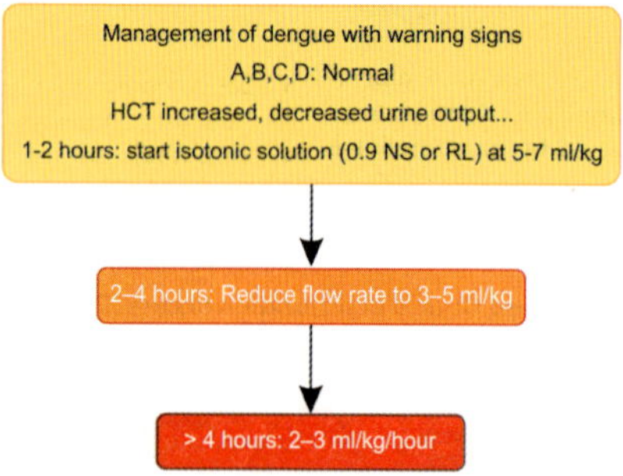

Figure 17: Management of dengue with warning signs.

SEVERE DENGUE

Triage Questions

Mother reports that her child with fever is either lethargic, more sleepy than usual, not as usual or has inconsolable cry. She may also report history of breathlessness.

Management of Severe Dengue with Warning Signs with Compensated Shock

- Airway and breathing: Oxygen is provided using the Jackson-Rees circuit.
- Circulation: 0.9 NS is administered at 10 ml/kg @ 1 hour.
- Void urine or catheter is used to monitor hourly urine output.
- HCT is monitored after every fluid bolus.

RECOGNITION OF HYPOTENSIVE DENGUE (FIGURE 19)

History

Mother reports that her child with fever is not as usual or more sleepy, has inconsolable cry (if infant) or lethargic. She may also report that her child has breathlessness (check whether episodic or since birth to rule out asthma or congestive heart failure).

> *Compensated shock may take hours to develop. When hypotension ensues, cardiac arrest occurs in minutes.*

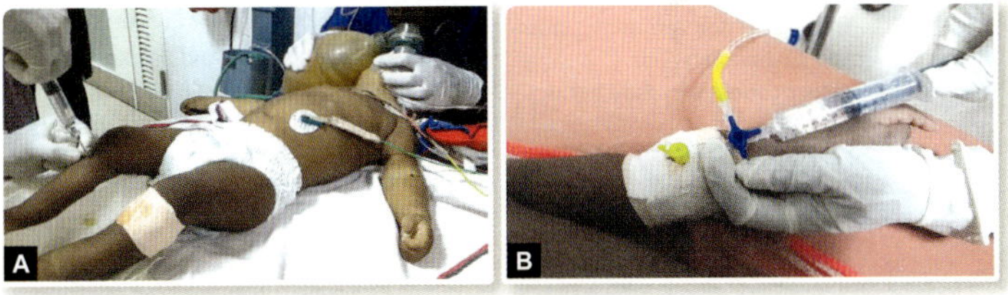

Figures 18A and B: Airway is opened using the head tilt, chin lift maneuver. BVM ventilation is initiated. Fluids are rushed via IO or using pull push method.

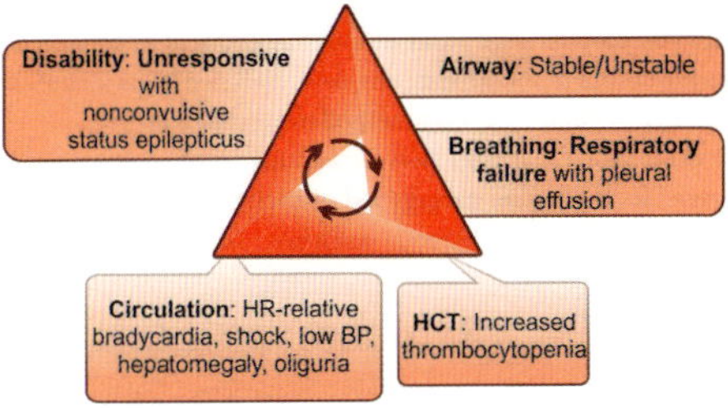

Figure 19: Physiological status: Airway unstable; Breathing: Respiratory distress; Circulation: Relative bradycardia, cardiogenic hypotensive shock; Disability: Altered level of consciousness with NCSE.

Management of Hypotensive Dengue (Fig. 21)

- Oxygen is provided using a Jackson-Rees circuit or noninvasive ventilation via BIPAP machine if the child has respiratory distress. If apneic initiate BVM ventilation.
- Intubation is ideally avoided due to risk of bleeding.
- Vascular access is obtained and 10-20 mL/kg NS is rushed rapidly using pull-push technique.
- Blood is withdrawn for grouping, cross-matching and lab investigations.
- Check hematocrit after every fluid bolus.
- Urinary catheter is inserted to monitor hourly urine output. Aim for urine output of 1 mL/kg/hour.

  If shock refractory to 20 L/kg crystalloid/colloid following must be considered:
- Fall in hematocrit or hypotension: Plan 5-10 mL/kg of fresh (less than 72 hours old) whole blood.
- Call for Epinephrine infusion @ (3-1 mcg/kg/minute).
- Metabolic abnormalities are corrected.
- GNS with potassium and calcium are initiated at maintenance rates.

Table 4: Fluids in hypotensive shock. If BP remains low, epinephrine infusion is initiated along with fluids.

HCT increasing with no improvement	HCT stable with improvement
• Second bolus of colloid of 10–20 mL/kg over 30 minutes–1 hour • If shock persists with high HCT colloid 3rd bolus 10–20 mL/kg over 1 hour • If shock persists and HCT remains high, start inotropes	• Reduce colloid to 7–10 mL/kg over 1–2 hours, then reduce to crystalloid

KEY POINTS

1. Repeated rapid cardiopulmonary and cerebral assessment in conjunction with hematological and urine output monitoring during defervescence helps identify the critical phase.
2. Adequate shock correction is the best method to prevent bleeding.
3. Noninvasive ventilation or Jackson-Rees circuit aids oxygen delivery with CPAP. The latter, reduces the need for intubation during fluid resuscitation in dengue.

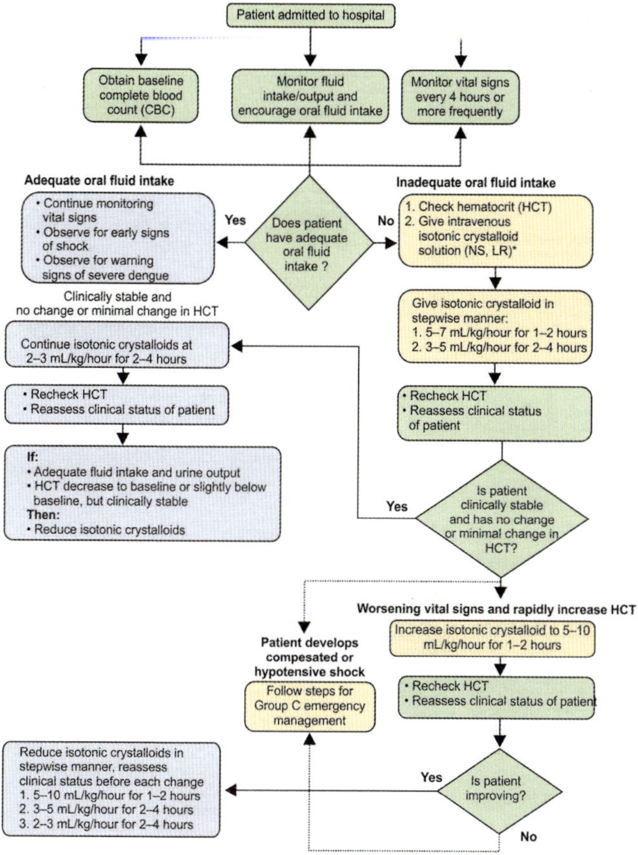

Figure 20: Management of severe dengue with compensated shock (*Source:* Handbook for clinical management of dengue, 2012).

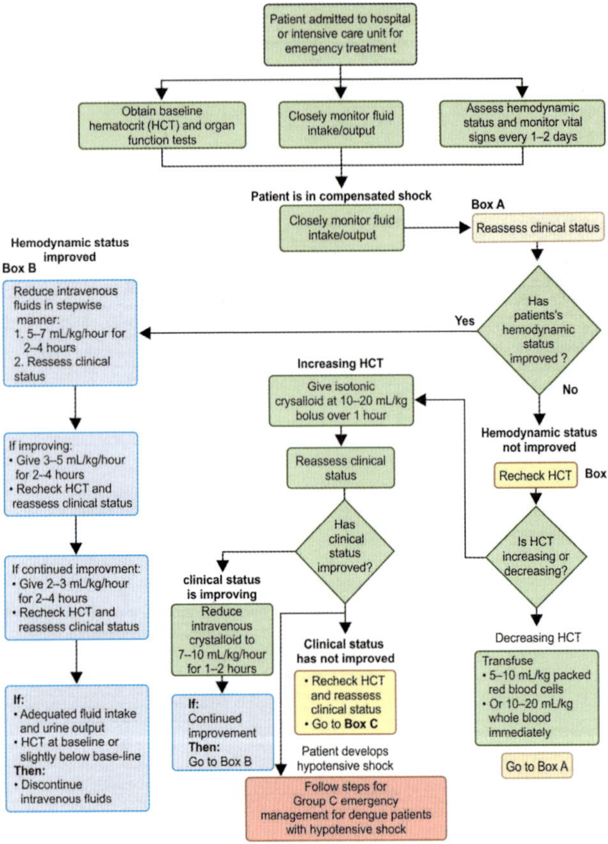

Figure 21: Management of severe dengue with hypotensive shock (Source: WHO Handbook for Clinical Management of Dengue, 2012).

ANAPHYLACTIC SHOCK

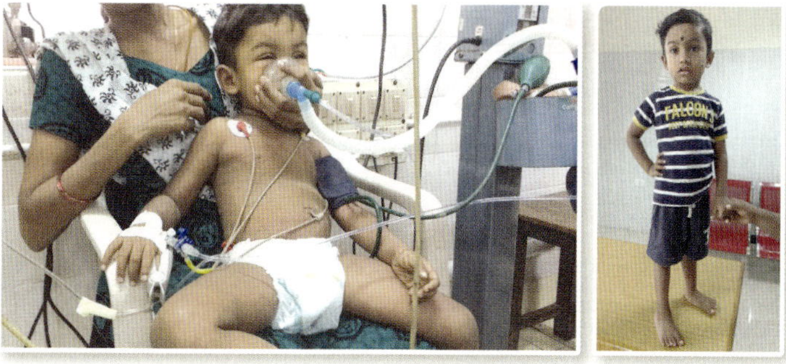

This picture shows a child being managed for anaphylactic shock, with the JR circuit, large volume fluids and epinephrine infusion. Note the giant urticaria and angioedema.

PATHOPHYSIOLOGY (FIGURE 22)

Anaphylactic shock is defined as an acute clinical syndrome caused by exposure to a foreign substance to which the patient has been previously sensitized. It is defined as a severe, life-threatening, generalized or systemic hypersensitivity reaction.

Airway

- Edema of the airway results in lethal airway obstruction (stridor).

Breathing

- Bronchospasm (respiratory distress with wheeze).

Circulation

- Sudden and severe vasodilation contributes to relative hypovolemia.
- Increased vascular permeability results in absolute hypovolemia.
- The resultant profound loss of effective circulating volume leads to sudden cardiovascular collapse the commonest prearrest manifestation.
- Swelling develops over skin of face and mouth. mucosa of the mouth, throat and tongue and hands.
- The swelling can be itchy or painful.
- Urticaria may develop concurrently

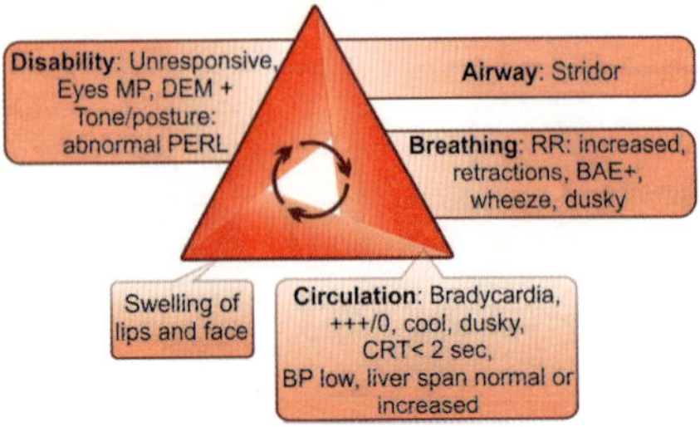

Figure 22: Anaphylactic shock

Airway: Stridor; Breathing: Respiratory distress; Circulation: Hypotensive shock.
Disability: Altered level of consciousness.

PRE-HOSPITAL CARE

- Remove allergen if possible (such as insect parts)
- Advice patients with stridor or respiratory distress to adopt a position of airway comfort
- If victim is feeling faint or unable to sit or stand, advice him to lie down
- Hypotensive patients can rapidly progress to cardiac arrest, if they are in the upright position.
- Place unresponsive children, who are breathing in the recovery position (on their side).

MANAGEMENT IN THE ED

Airway and Breathing

- Provide oxygen using Jackson-Rees
- Plan early intubation
- Rapid, progressive edema can obscure all landmarks, making bag-valve-mask ventilation difficult
- Avoid paralytic agents
- Smaller endotracheal tubes should be available.

Circulation

- Secure vascular access and administer isotonic fluid boluses.
- 60–200 mL/kg of isotonic fluids may be needed to restore peripheral perfusion and blood pressure.

> *Epinephrine is administered @ 0.1 mg/kg per dose (1: 1000)* **DEEP IM** *at 5 minute intervals based on patient's response.*

- Perform the rapid cardiopulmonary cerebral assessment following each bolus to determine whether the child is showing signs of improvement, deterioration or is remaining status quo.

- If bradycardia or hypotensive shock occurs, initiate epinephrine infusion @ 1–4 mcg/kg/minute.

Intramuscular adrenaline should be given as early as possible after the onset of anaphylaxis.

An alpha-receptor agonist, it reverses peripheral vasodilation and reduces edema. Its beta-receptor activity dilates the bronchial airways, increases the force of myocardial contraction, and suppresses histamine and leukotriene release.

Beta-2 adrenergic receptors also exist on mast cells. Adrenaline acts on these receptors, thereby inhibiting degranulation, and reducing the severity of IgE mediated allergic reactions.

SQ or inhaled routes for adrenaline not recommended for the treatment of an anaphylactic reaction because absorption is inadequate.

Though arrhythmias are uncommon in children with anaphylaxis, when epinephrine is being administered, cardiac rhythm should be monitored.

Age appropriate dose of injection Adrenaline or Epinephrine

- 12 years: 500 μg IM (0.5 mL), i.e. same as adult dose, 300 μg (0.3 mL), if child is small or prepubertal
- 6–12 years: 300 μg IM (0.3 mL)
- 6 months–6 years: 150 μg IM (0.15 mL)
- < 6 months: 150 μg IM (0.15 mL)

Antihistamines

- H1-antihistamine helps to counter histamine-mediated vasodilation and bronchoconstriction.
- Administer chlorpheniramine maleate intramuscularly or slowly through the intravenous route.

Injection Chlorphenaramine maleate

- > 12 years and adults: 10 mg IM or IV slowly
- > 6–12 years: 5 mg IM or IV slowly
- > 6 months–6 years: 2.5 mg IM or IV slowly
- < 6 months: 250 μg/kg IM or IV slowly.

Steroids

Steroids reduces duration of illness.

Injection Hydrocortisone

- > 12 years and adults: 200 mg IM or IV slowly
- > 6–12 years: 100 mg IM or IV slowly
- > 6 months–6 years: 50 mg IM or IV slowly
- < 6 months: 25 mg IM or IV slowly.

KEY POINTS

1. Epinephrine is the drug of choice in anaphylactic shock.
2. Epinephrine is given deep intramuscular.
3. Large volume of isotonic fluids are needed to resolve shock due to anaphylaxis.

OBSTRUCTIVE SHOCK

Obstructive Shock due to Pneumothorax or Empyema

1. Recognize right sided pneumothorax clinically when upper border of liver dullness is obliterated by resonant percussion note.
2. Recognize empyema or pleural effusion when upper border of liver dullness is obliterated by stony dullness
3. Anticipate pneumothorax as cause of shock in poly trauma victims

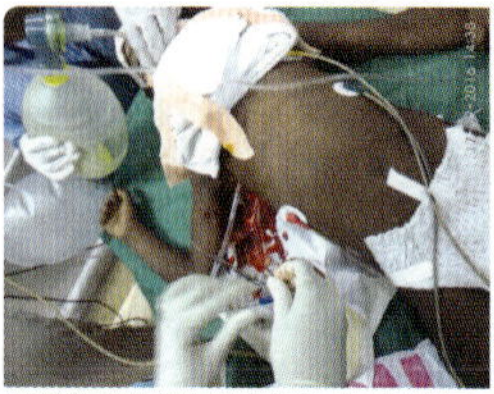

Figure 23: Thoracotomy for hemopneumothorax (Call surgeon for help).

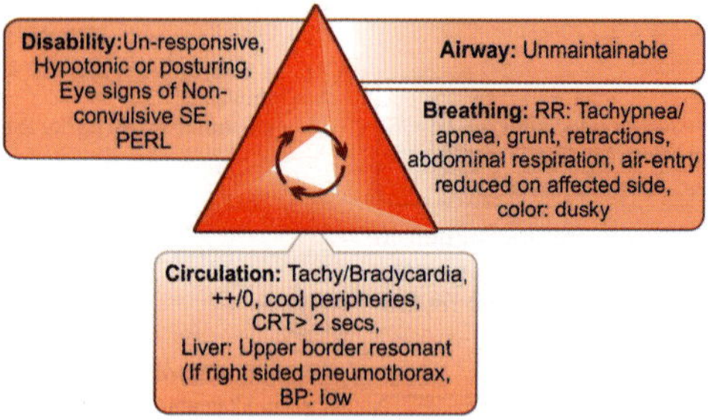

Figure 24: A: Unstable; **B:** Respiratory distress or respiratory failure; **C:** Hypotensive shock with obliteration of liver dullness (responance is suggestive of pneumothorax); **D:** ALOC/NCSE.

4. If obstructive shock is due to embyema or hemothorax (Figures 23 and 24) large volume fluids may be needed (septic shock). If obstructive shock occurs due to congenited diapharagmatic hornia or cardiac tamponade, less than 20 mL/kg may be warranted.
5. Shock secondary to pneumothorax or empyema will resolve only when obstruction is relieved by thoracocentesis followed by thoracotomy.

Obstructive Shock due to Empyema or Hemothorax (Figure 25)

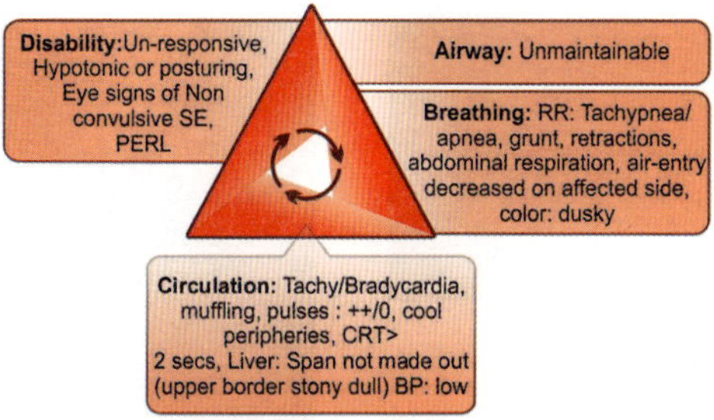

Figure 25: A: Unstable; **B:** Respiratory distress or respiratory failure; **C:** Hypotensive shock with obliteration of liver dullness (stony dull indicates pleural fluid); **D:** ALOC/NCSE

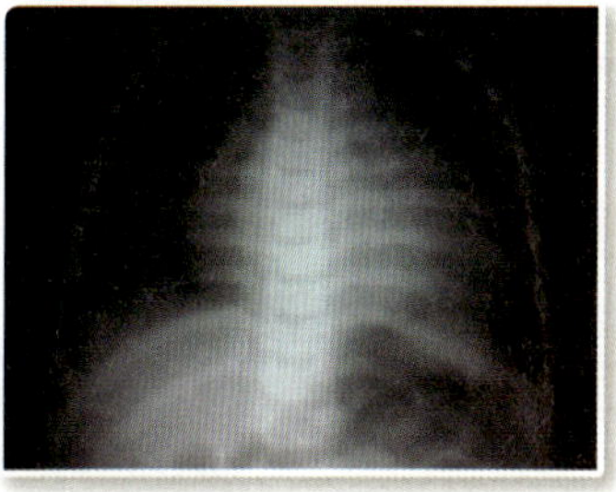

Massive pericardial effusion.

Tension pneumothorax, massive empyema, cardiac tamponade are some of the causes of obstruction to cardiac output. Needle thoracocentesis or pericardiocentesis is necessary to relieve obstruction to cardiac output.

Obstructive shock will not completely resolve with fluids, inotropes and intubation. Rapid relief of obstruction to cardiac output is therapeutic.

1. Suspect, when respiratory failure, is associated with muffled heart sounds, shock, hepatomegaly, low BP
2. Ultrasound and chest X-ray are diagnostic

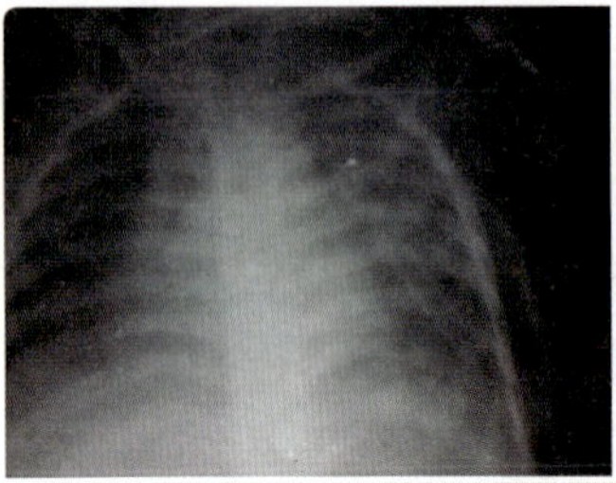

Note the drainage tube in the pericardium. Pericardiocentesis in the ED, relieves shock due to obstruction to cardiac output (Call for surgeon or senior for help).

3. Pericardiocentesis is essential to resolve shock due to cardiac tamponade.

Figure 26 shows the child following pericardiocentesis (X-rays shown above).

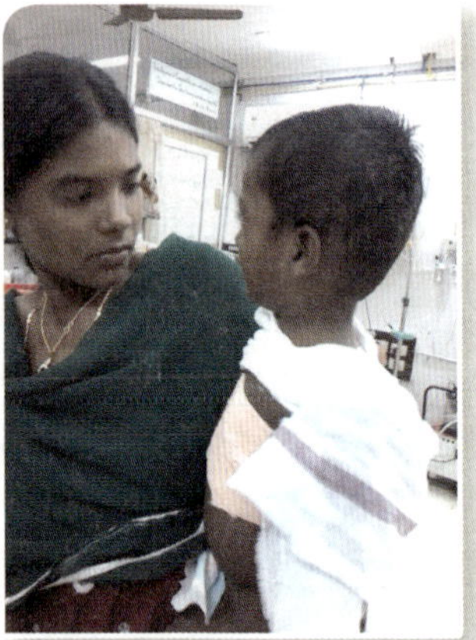

Figure 26: Post-pericardiectomy

INTRAOSSEOUS ACCESS

SETTING UP AN INTRAOSSEOUS ACCESS TRAY (FIGURE 26)

1. Sand bag
2. Stainless steel tray, cups with gauze, which can be autoclaved.
3. Bone marrow needle (14 gauge) with trocar
4. Prefilled syringes
5. Betadine, tincture Benzoin
6. Dynaplast (cut to fix the needle)
7. Hole towel
8. Gloves
9. 3-way adapter, infusion set.

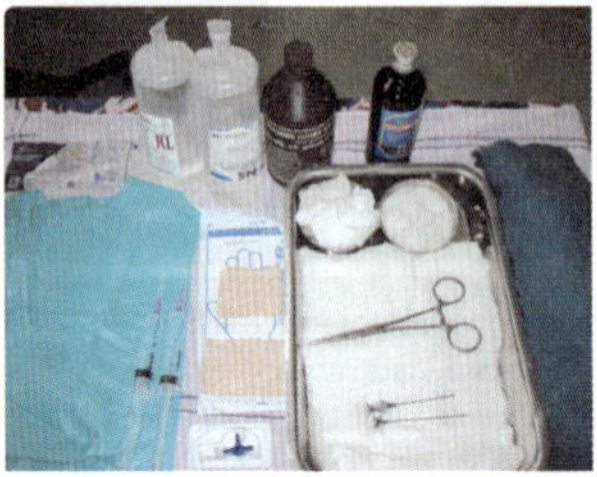

Figure 27: Intraosseous tray.

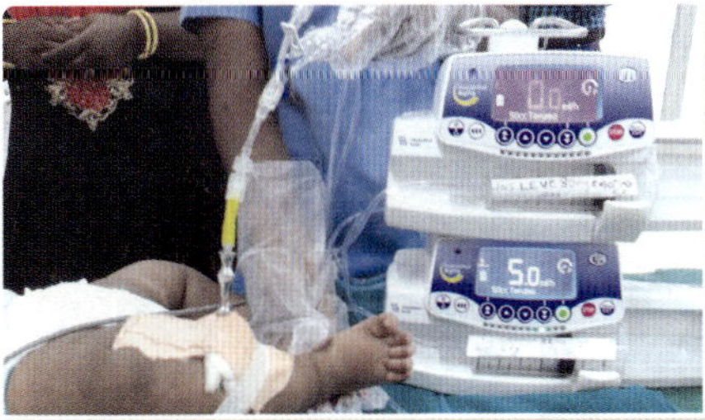

The picture shows a 3-way being used to infuse, fluids, Dopamine and levetiracetam via a single IO access.

POSITIONING AND METHOD OF INSERTION OF IO NEEDLE

- Place a sand bag under the knee.
- Externally rotate and abduct the knee.
- Identify tibial tubercle.
- The point of insertion is 1 cm below and medial to the tibial tubercle (Figure 28).

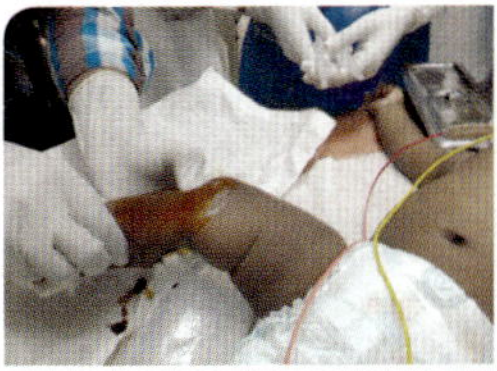

Figure 28: Identify point of entry by using the tibial tubercle as land mark

Intraosseous access may be removed once a peripheral venous access is obtained. In the management of severe shock, IO is retained even, if a peripheral IV line is obtained later. While, the peripheral IV access is useful for administration of fluid boluses, anticonvulsants, anesthetic medications, dextrose, etc. during resuscitation, the IO line may be used exclusively for inotrope infusion.

OTHER SITES OF IO INSERTION (FIGURES 29 TO 36)

1. Medial malleolus and medial end of femur

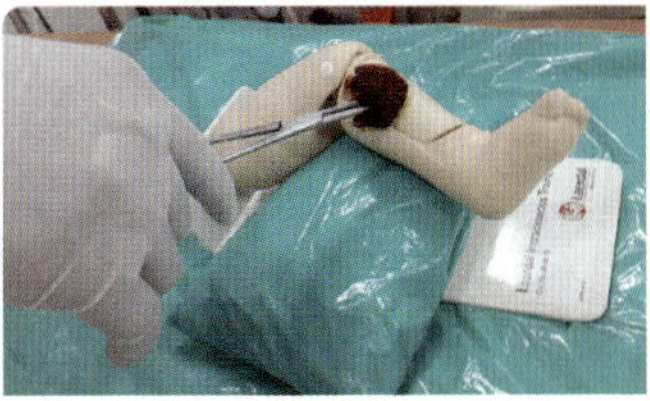

Figure 29: Clean the site of insertion with Betadine-soaked gauze.

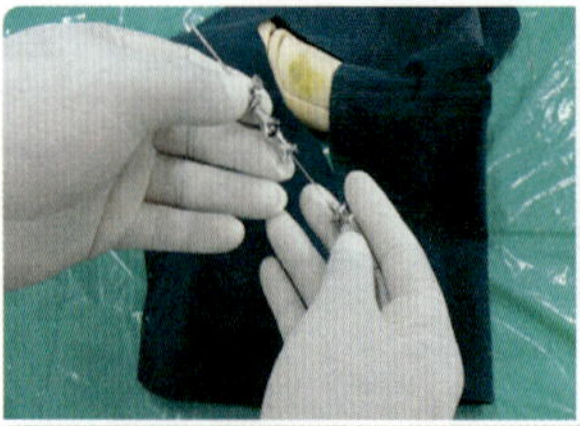

Figure 30: The bone marrow aspiration needle (14-16 G) can be used as intraosseous needle. The trocar is useful in preventing the needle from getting clogged by marrow particles.

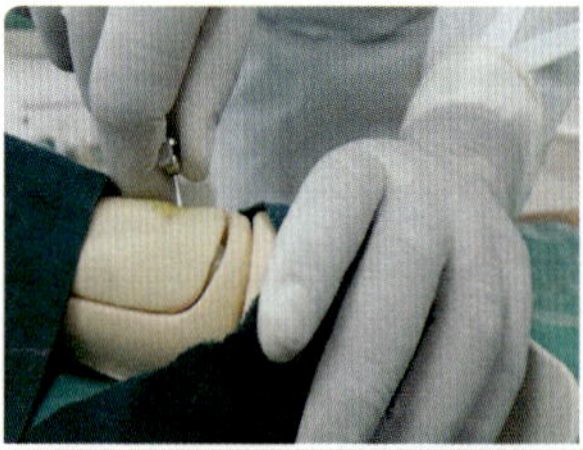

Figure 31: Use thumb of the left hand to fix the tibial tuberosity to guide insertion of the bone marrow needle. Use screwing movements to introduce the bone marrow needle into the tibia. Enter the tibia perpendicular to its shaft. Continue to fix the knee with the left hand. The BM needle is introduced until a "give" is felt.

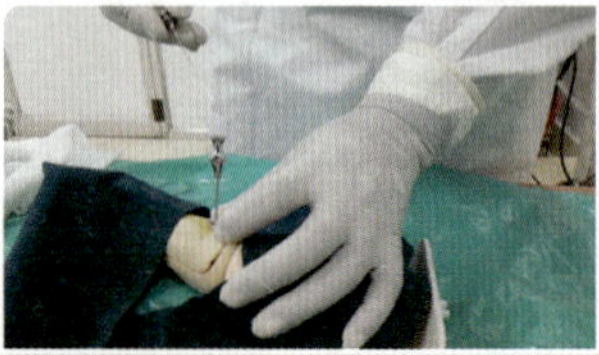

Figure 32: The needle will stand proud. The trocar is removed. Prior to insertion of bone marrow needle, prefilled syringe should be available. Connect the syringe to the bone marrow needle and manually push fluid.

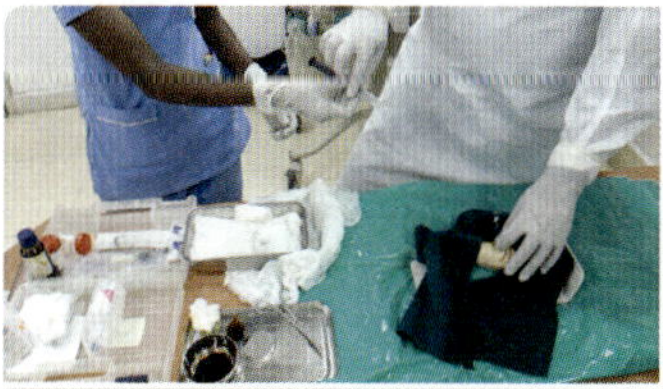

Figure 33: The fluid-filled syringe should be prepared concurrently during IO access. Waiting to fill the syringe after entry will delay infusion and result in clogging of the needle with marrow. Fixing the needle with the left hand, the fluid is pushed through the needle.

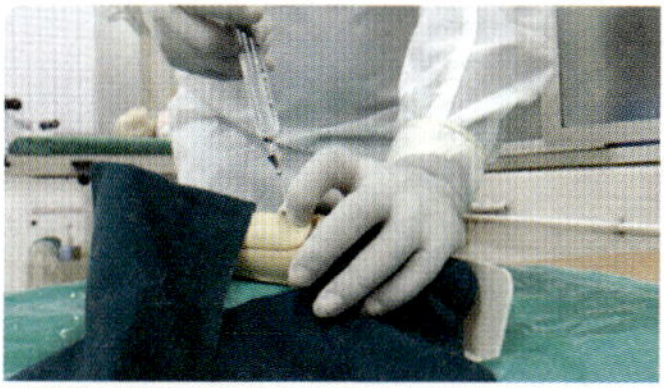

Figure 34: Effort is needed to push the fluid into the marrow space. Intraosseous (IO) access is a rapid, safe and effective route for administration of fluids, epinephrine, anticonvulsants, blood products and inotropes. Onset of action and drug levels are comparable to venous administration. Administration of a drug should be followed by a 5 ml saline flush to promote entry into the central circulation.

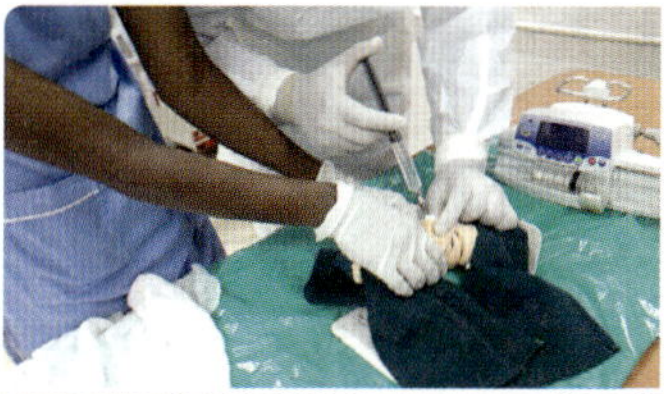

Figure 35: During bolus therapy, dislodgement of the IO needle can occur resulting in extravasation. To avoid this complication fix the needle with gauze and dynaplast.

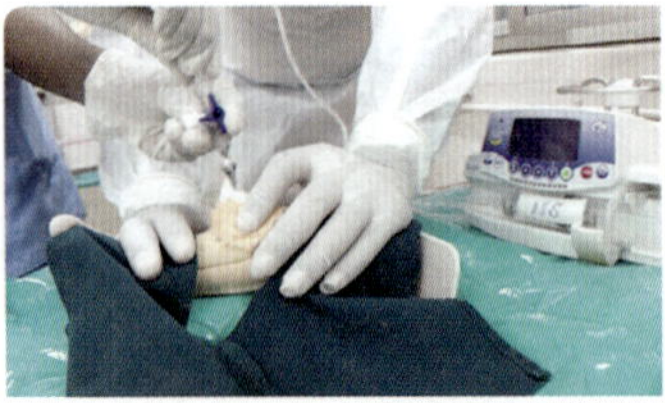

Figure 36: Fluids will not run freely from the intravenous bottle. An infusion pump may be needed to push fluid under pressure. Usually, a second peripheral IV line is obtained after the first bolus through the IO line. A 3-way device, aids in administering more than one infusion via the IO line.

KEY POINTS

1. If intravenous access is not obtained after 2 attempts or 90 seconds, secure an intraosseous access.
2. Use "screwing" movements. Avoid pushing the needle directly into the bone.
3. Fixing the IO needle is crucial. Bolus therapy can lead to dislodgement of the IO needle.
4. Avoid using blood set needles or needles that lack a trocar.

Protocol 6.3: PEMC approach: Management of shock with or without myocardial dysfunction

APPEARANCE: Incessant cry, lethargy, not recognizing mother, sleepy, fighting mask, not able to walk, floppy, agitated, combative, talking irrelevantly, posturing, GTC, eye deviation, nystagmus, lid twitch (NCSE signals severe hypoxia/shock) PERL

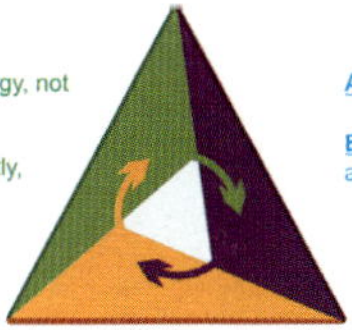

AIRWAY: Maintainable/stridor/not maintainable

BREATHING: RR ↑ ↓, grunt +/-, retractions +/-, abdominal respiration, added sounds

CIRCULATION: HR ↑ ↓, CRT > 2 sec, difficult/bounding to feel dorsalis, abnormal color, warm/cool peripheries, BP ↑ ↓, liver span: N/hepatomegaly

Assess after first 20 mL/kg bolus; 1. Further boluses based on etiology; 2. Response to therapy:

1. Shock goals achieved → Shift to ward, monitor closely for recurrence of shock

2. Shock goals not achieved
No PE/hepatomegaly →
1. If sepsis/hypovolemia/anaphylaxis: continue boluses
2. If not stop fluids, initiate inotrope

3. Shock goals not achieved
/features of PE+ →
1. Stop fluid/initiate inotrope, CPAP/ET
2. PE/hepatomegaly resolve, shock persists
3. ? Sepsis: continue fluid boluses
? Hypovolemia: continue boluses
4. If no sepsis, hypovolemia, anaphylaxis: no further fluids

Etiology: Sepsis, hypovolemia, anaphylaxis: 40–120 mL/kg in initial hours of resuscitation
Asthma, status epilepticus: Fluid requirement additional 10 mL/kg (max 20–30 mL/kg) if still in shock, further fluids warranted only if history of vomiting, sepsis, anaphylaxis
Envenomation, submersion injury: If shock persists after initial volume, inotrope infusion, early intubation with PEEP
Trauma: 10 mL/kg aliquots, control bleeding and if shock not responsive to 50 mL/kg consider blood transfusion and surgical exploration
Isolated closed head trauma, tension pneumothorax cardiac tamponade: 20 mL/kg
Cardiogenic shock: CHD, myocarditis: max fluid up to 20 mL/kg in aliquots of 5–10 mL/kg, early intubation to provide PEEP, inotrope infusion
DKA: 10–20 mL/kg over 1–2 hour

Treat etiology simultaneously:
- Antibiotics, source control in sepsis
- Bronchodilators for asthma
- Anticonvulsant therapy for seizures
- Antidotes, antivenins for toxins, envenomation
- Cardioversion/adenosine in SVT
- Thoracocentesis: pneumothorax
- Control bleed: Trauma

Each step in the management of shock is guided by repeated rapid cardiopulmonary assessment. These are broad guidelines and treatment should be individualized for the patient at hand.

7
CHAPTER

Disability

Chapter Outline

- Altered level of consciousness.
- Generalized tonic-clonic seizures
- Status epilepticus: Convulsive and subtle status epilepticus

DEFINITION

Consciousness is the state of full awareness of self and one's relationship to the environment. Based on severity, impairment of consciousness is described as obtundation, stupor or coma (Figure 1).

The study from the UK reported that if the Glasgow Coma Scale (GCS) was less than 12 in children between 1 month and 18 years of age for greater than 6 hours, mortality was as high as 40%.

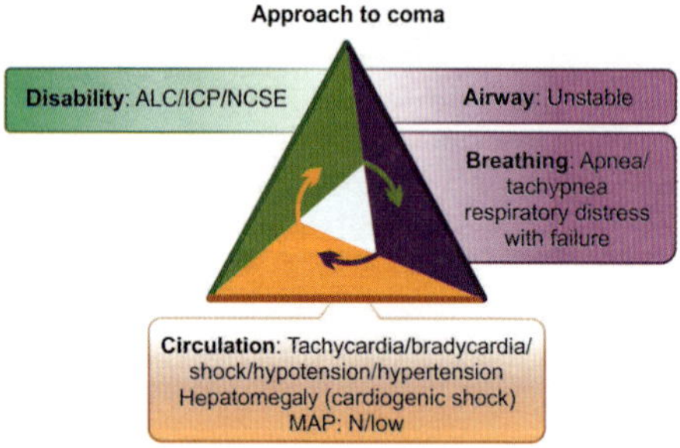

Figure 1: Using the pediatric assessment triangle to evaluate coma.

- **Airway:** Open the airway using head tilt and chin lift maneuver (Figure 2)

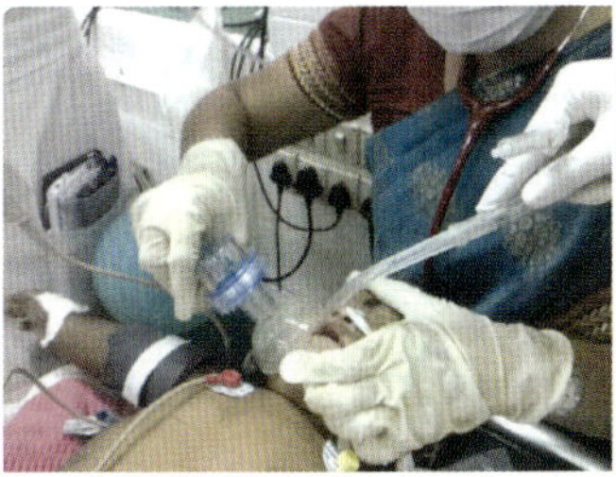

Figure 2: Head tilt chin lift

- Suction oropharyngeal secretions (Figure 3)
- Nasogastric decompression

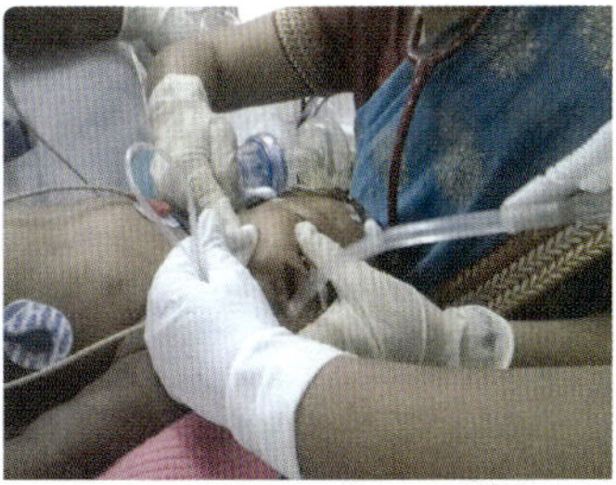

Figure 3: Suction oro-pharynx using yankouver suction tip after turning head to one side. Note the naso-gastric tube held in the left hand of the nurse, ready for introduction.

- Initiate bag valve mask ventilation if ineffective respirations are noted (Figure 4)

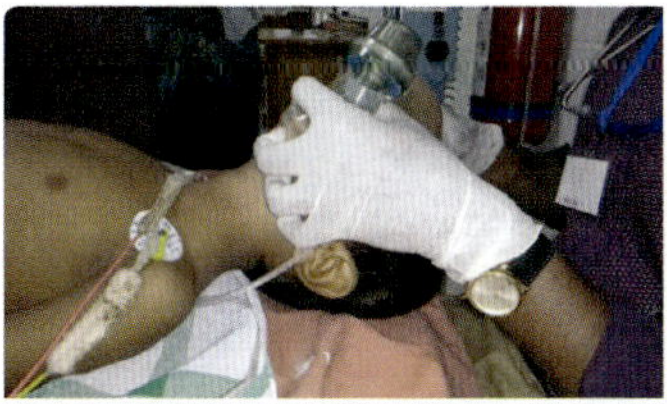

Figure 4: Presume that every un-responsive child, is potentially apneic on arrival. Plan to start bag valve mask ventilation.

- Apply Jackson-Rees circuit, if spontaneously breathing (Figure 5)

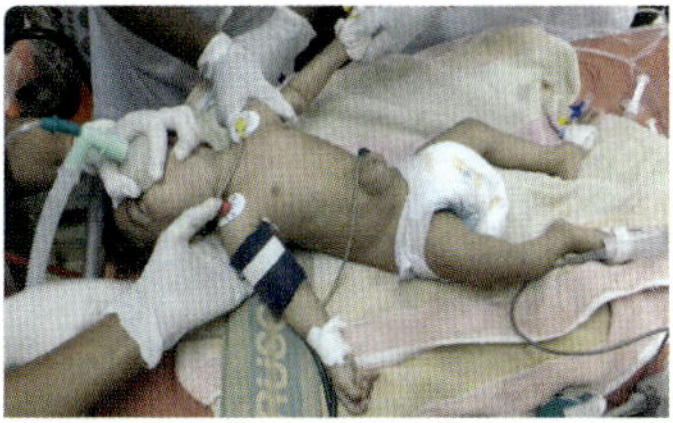

Figure 5: If crying (airway stable), and spontaneous breathing is noted, provide oxygen via the JR circuit.

Loss of tone of the oro-pharyngeal muscles causes falling back of the tongue resulting in airway obstruction. Loss of cough or swallowing reflexes lead to pooling of secretions. Airway obstruction, worsen underlying hypoxia, shock, cardiac failure, status epilepticus and ICP. Plan to intubate. Call for anesthetist. Anesthetic drugs are essential to avoid aggravating intracranial pressure.

- If coma is due to shock due to sepsis, hypovolemia or anaphylaxis, plan for 60–80 mL/kg NS. Monitor for signs of pulmonary edema during fluid resuscitation.
- If coma is due to head trauma, envenomation, submersion or cardiac causes restrict to 10-20 mL/kg) (Figure 6).

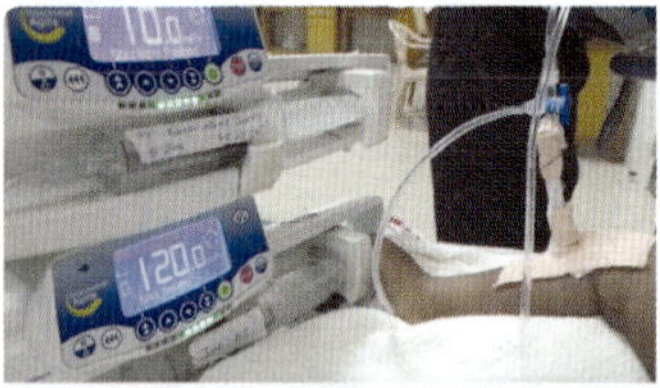

Figure 6: Administering NS if signs of shock are noted.

- Check dextrostix and give 25% dextrose (2 ml/kg), if blood sugar is less than 60 mg/dl
- Administer injection lorazepam, if eye lid twitch or conjugate deviation or nystagmus (subtle status epilepticus) is noted (0.1 mg/kg) (Figure 7).

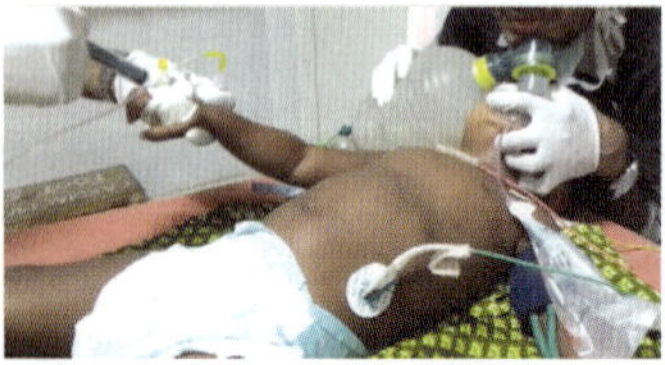

Figure 7: Administration of lorazepam if signs of GTCs or eye signs of SE are noted

As resuscitation is in progress, look for:

a. Evidence of trauma
b. Evidence of acute or chronic systemic illness
c. Evidence of drug ingestion (history of spilled or missing tablets)
d. Bite marks (snake envenomation)

- Check electrolytes.
    i. Ionized calcium is less than 1 mmol/dl, administer 0.5–1 ml/kg of 10% calcium gluconate.
    ii. Serum sodium less than 115 mmol/dl, administer 5 ml/kg of 3% NS over 5–10 minutes
- Catheterize and monitor urine output
- Collect blood for complete blood count, coagulation screen, blood culture (if febrile), liver function tests, plasma ammonia, plasma lactate.
- Plasma and urine for toxicology, organic and amino acids should be sent in appropriate cases.
- Avoid LP if abnormal breathing patterns, shock, bradycardia, hypertension, GCS < 8, convulsive or non-convulsive status epilepticus, abnormal dolls eye movement, dilated pupils, abnormal posture and ICP. Delay LP and treat empirically when in doubt.
- Initiate antibiotics, artesunate and acyclovir while awaiting culture and PCR reports.
- Cranial CT, is considered only after resuscitation is complete.

While the A and B are being managed, ask focused history. Life saving interventions precede history taking:

1. Unresponsiveness associated with fits? posturing? upward gaze?

2. Time? Place: Where was it noted?
3. Regained basal consciousness?
4. Any precipitating event (diarrhea, vomiting, breathlessness, allergens, trauma, toxin?)
5. Drop in mental status between the event and now?
6. Normal development?
7. Co-morbidities?
8. Drugs?
9. Pre-hospital care?

ICP (Figures 8A and B)

Nurse the child in the 30° head up position.

- Keep head in neutral position to avoid kinking of the neck.
- Avoid noxious stimuli. Take efforts to provide pain relief and sedation during painful procedures.
- Maintain euglycemia.
- Control fever aggressively.
- Treat seizures.
- Administer an antibiotic (Ceftriaxone) empirically, if sepsis is suspected.
- Hyperosmolar therapy: Infuse 3% saline (5 mL/Kg) followed by continuous infusion between 0.1 and 1.0 mL/kg/h.
- Ventilate to maintain eucapnia ($PaCO_2$: 35–40 mm Hg).

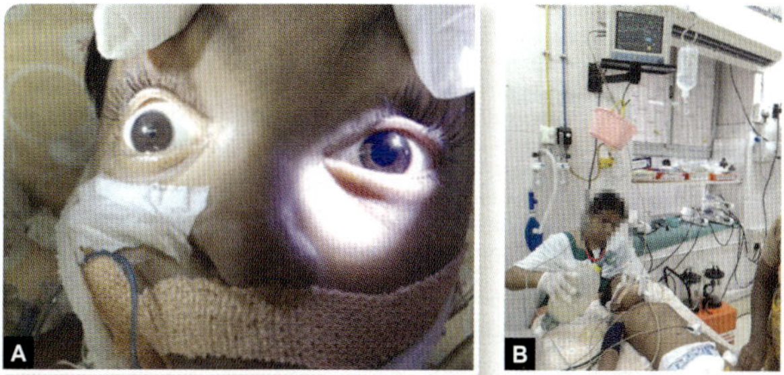

Figures 8A and B: (A) Unequal pupils in comatose child; (B) Unresponsive child who has been intubated, corrected for shock and ICP. Note bradycardia on the monitor.

KEY POINTS

1. Correction of hypoxia, shock, nonconvulsive status epilepticus and hypoglycemia improves survival in comatose victims.
2. If malaria, scrub, leptospirosis, HINI, or herpes simplex is suspected, the appropriate antimicrobial drug should be infused.
3. Anticipate ICP and treat appropriately, if coma persists despite correction of hypoxia, shock, NCSE and metabolic parameters.
4. Shock management is not a contraindication in children with ICP.

GENERALIZED TONIC-CLONIC SEIZURES AND STATUS EPILEPTICUS

Generalized tonic-clonic seizures (GTCSs) are characterized by a sudden onset of tonic, clonic movements of voluntary muscles. In addition, the child also loses consciousness and is unable to maintain tone and posture.

Sudden unresponsiveness with loss of tone and posture in an alert child (without precipitating event): Suspect subtle status epilepticus.

The loss of internal tone and posture of the palatepharyngeal muscles and the tongue is far more dangerous. The tongue falls back, obstructing the airway (the passage that connects the oropharynx and the larynx), thereby preventing the child from breathing. Unresponsiveness also results in inability to cough (a protective reflex that prevents secretions from entering the lung) and pooling of secretions. The larynx (also voluntary or skeletal muscles) can convulse, further aggravating airway obstruction.

Whilst the tonic-clonic movements of the limbs look alarming, it is the seizure activity of the intercostal muscles that prevent the child from breathing effectively, that is truly dangerous!

GTCSs are dangerous not because of the tonic-clonic movements of the limbs but because the air passage is obstructed and the child is not able to breathe effectively during the event.

Fortunately, majority of GTCs resolve within 2 minutes.

Definition

Status epilepticus (SE) is defined when GTCSs persist for more than 5 minutes in children > 5 years of age or two or more seizures occur consecutively without an intervening period of full recovery of consciousness. Overt generalized SE, if left untreated, will evolve into subtle SE.

Pathophysiology

SE, a primarily hypoxic event, can also lead to cardiac dysfunction, pulmonary edema and shock. If not controlled urgently, ongoing SE, can cause vasodilatation and capillary leak in the systemic circulation. The capillary leak in the pulmonary circulation leads to acute lung injury. Established SE (SE lasting for more than 30 minutes can lead to heart failure).

The failing heart and leaky pulmonary capillaries result in pulmonary edema (Figures 9A and B).

Cardiogenic or noncardiogenic pulmonary edema and shock are common in children presenting with established SE!

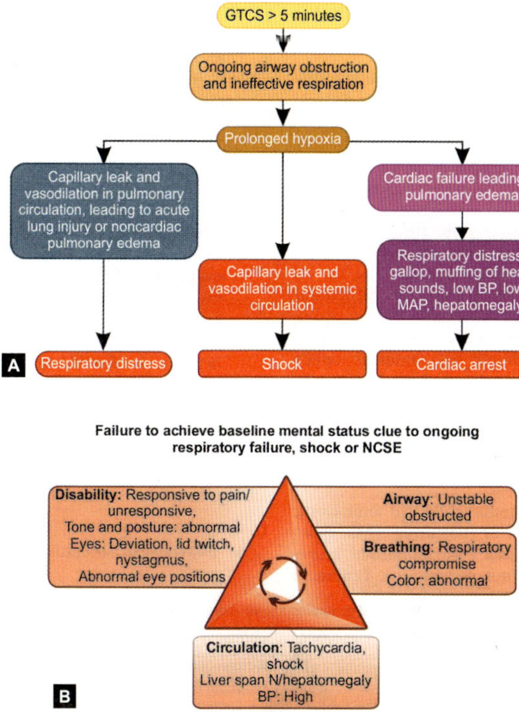

Figures 9A and B: (A) Pathophysiology of shock and cardiac dysfunction due to status epilepticus; (B) Complications of uncontrolled generalized tonic-clonic convulsions.

The initial priority in the management of GTCs is focused on resolving hypoxia.

Prehospital Therapy

- Place the convulsing child on his side, (recovery position) to enable drainage of secretions.

- Open the airway using the head tilt chin lift maneuver (while maintaining the recovery position).
- Suction the airway. Avoid stimulating the posterior pharyngeal wall since it could cause vagal-induced bradycardia.
- Provide oxygen with a non-rebreather mask.
- If not breathing, initiate bag valve mask ventilation.
- Correct shock with 10–20 mL/kg of normal saline or Ringer's lactate.
- Administer Midazolam (0.2 mg/kg) via the intramuscular or intrabuccal or intranasal route.
- Fever, a common cause of seizures in children, should be controlled rapidly by tepid sponging and placing a rectal suppository of paracetamol.

Focused history that should be elicited when a child is brought with abnormal neurological movements associated with unresponsiveness.

1. Confirm whether child had tonic clonic movements or posturing (Ask mom to demonstrate). All abnormal movements are not convulsions. Failure to differentiate between fits and posturing can lead to wrong treatment and death.
2. Find out time and place. This question aids in determining the approximate duration of hypoxia and shock.
3. Ask whether the child has regained basal consciousness (if not regained, anticipate NCSE)
4. a. Ask whether fever, diarrhea, breathlessness, trauma or toxin preceded these movements.
   b. Find out, whether, these precipitating events were followed by progressive loss of consciousness between the event and the GTCs (if yes, anticipate that the GTCs are secondary to hypoxia, shock or trauma).
5. Find out whether
   i. Is development normal or not?
   ii. Comorbid conditions?
   iii. Prehospital care?

Emergency Department (Figure 10)

1. Oxygen is provided via:
   a. BVM device, if the child presents with apnea and shock.

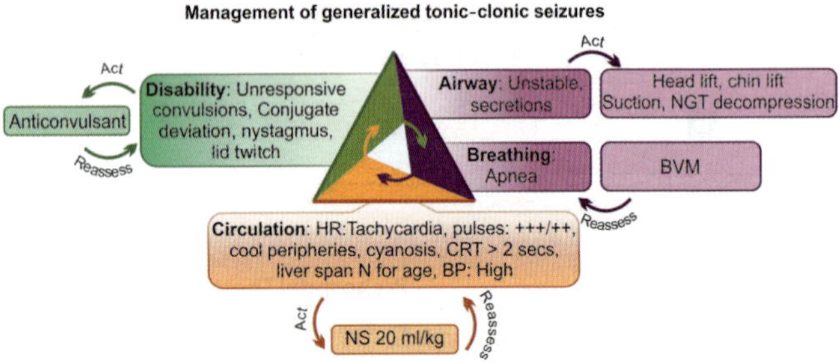

Figure 10: Management of generalized tonic-clonic seizures.

b. Jackson-Rees circuit to provide CPAP, if the child presents with respiratory distress or develops respiratory distress during the management of shock.
2. 10–20 mL/kg of NS boluses is infused over 10–20 minutes until shock is corrected.
3. If signs of pulmonary edema are un-masked during shock management, fluids are interrupted and an inotrope is infused. The choice of inotrope is based on the blood pressure.
   a. If BP is normal: Dopamine
   b. If BP is high: Dobutamine
   c. If BP is low: Epinephrine.

   Ongoing seizure activity results in loss of the protective (fit-stopping) effects mediated by GABA. At the same time, continued seizure activity results in mobilization of (fit-increasing) excitatory N-methyl-d-aspartate receptors. The reduced activity of GABA (seizure-stopping neuropeptides) and increased activity of N-methyl-d-aspartate receptors (seizure-provoking neuropeptides) result in a continuing SE.
4. Dextrostix should be used to measure sugar levels early in the management of SE. Documented hypoglycemia is corrected with an intravenous bolus of 2 mL/kg of 25% dextrose solution. Correct documented hypocalcemia.
5. Anticonvulsants (Table 1).

> *Treat until therapeutic goal of hypoxia, shock, cardiac dysfunction and subtle statue epilepticus is resolved (Figure 11).*

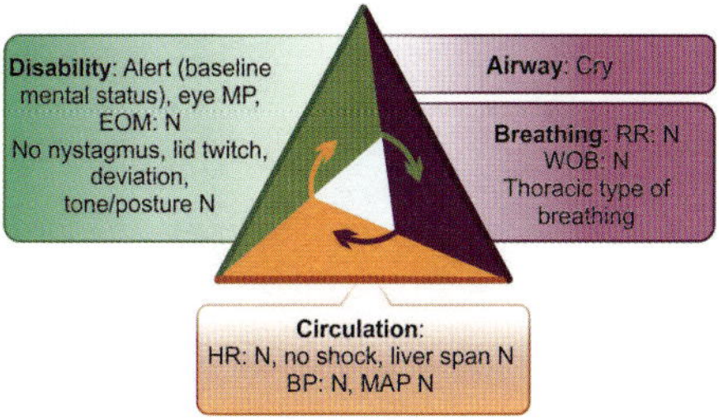

Figure 11: Therapeutic goals of status epilepticus resolution.

Table 1: Drugs used in emergency room for management of status epilepticus.

Drug	Initial dose	Route	IV administration	Onset of action	Half life	Adverse effects
Lorazepam	0.05 mg 0.1 mg/kg Max: 4 mg	IV	IV 0.5 mg/kg Infusion: 0.01–0.1 mg/kg/hr	1–3 mins	Neonates–40 hrs Children–10 hrs	Sedation, hypotension, bradycardia, respiratory depression, hyperactivity
Diazepam	0.05–0.3 mg/kg Max: < 5 yr–5 mg > 5 yr–10 mg PR dose – 0.5 mg/kg	IV PR	0.1 mg/kg/min	1–3 mins	Neonates–50.95 hrs Infants: 40–50 hrs Children 15–20 hrs	Sedation, hypotension, bradycardia, respiratory depression, hyperactivity Thrombophlebitis
Midazolam	0.1–0.15 mg/kg Max: 0.15 mg/kg	IV PR	Infusion: 1 mg/kg/min to max of 24 mg/kg/min	1–5 mins	Neonates: 4–12 hrs Children: 3–4 hrs	Sedation, hypotension, bradycardia, respiratory depression, apnea, laryngospasm, hyperactivity
Phenytoin	15–20 mg/kg Max: 1 gm	IV	Slow IV over a period of 20 mins @ 1 mg/kg/min to max of 50 mg/kg/min Monitor heart rate and BP during administration. Infusion may be titrated to maintain baseline heart rate	10 mins after the infusion is over	7–24 hrs (first-order kinetics do not apply)	Tachyarrhythmia commonly seen during administration. Decreased infusion rate. Bradyarrhythmia, gallop, pulmonary edema, hypotension noted during infusion is suggestive of underlying myocardial depression

Contd...

Contd...

Drug	Initial dose	Route	IV administration	Onset of action	Half life	Adverse effects
						due to refractory status epilepticus, severe sepsis, etc. Stop PHT secure the airway and initiate phenobarbitone. Dysarthria, ataxia, sedation, thrombophlebitis, purple glove syndrome
Fosphenytoin	15–20 mg PE/kg	IV IM	3 mg PE/kg/min to max 150 mg PE/min	7 min convert to phenytoin	12–29 hrs (first-order kinetics do not apply)	Dysarthria, ataxia, sedation, hypotension, arrhythmia
Valproic acid	15–20 mg/kg Max: 25 mg/kg	IV	5 mg/kg/min Infusion: 1–4 mg/kg/hr	-	>2 mon 7–13 hrs 2–14 yrs – 4020 hrs.	Hypotension, cardiac arrhythmias, hepatitis, pancreatitis
Phenobarbitone	20–30 mg/kg	Iv	2 mg/kg/min (max 100 mg/min)			Respiratory depression, sedation, requires intubation

KEY POINTS

1. Bag-valve-mask ventilation is initiated when children present with convulsive status epilepticus.
2. Correct shock, if identified.
3. If signs of pulmonary edema are noted, initiate inotrope therapy.
4. Treat until the airway is established, breathing is normal, heart rate, perfusion and BP are normal, hepatomegaly is resolved and eye signs of subtle status epilepticus have also resolved.

Protocol 7.1: PEMC approach: Altered mental status and abnormal movements in a critically ill child

- GTCS > 5 min
- Not regained consciousness between 2 episodes

APPEARANCE
- Unresponsive
- GTCS +

BREATHING
Apnea

CIRCULATION
- Tachycardia
- Compesated shock ±

CONVULSIVE STATUS EPILEPTICUS

- Manage ABC
- Anticonvulsant drugs

- Sudden onset of unresponsiveness
- GTCS ±

APPEARANCE
- Unresponsive
- Tone abnormal
- Posture abnormal
- Eyelid twitching ±
- Nystagmus ±
- Conjugate deviation ±
- DEM defective
- No GTCS

BREATHING
Apnea

CIRCULATION
- Tachycardia
- Compensated shock ±

NON-CONVULSIVE STATUS EPILEPTICUS

- Manage ABC
- Anticonvulsant drugs

- Any illness
- Unresponsiveness

APPEARANCE
- Unresponsive
- Tone abnormal
- Posturing +
- DEM ±

BREATHING
- Bradypnea
- WOB ↓
- TV ↓
- Cyanosis +

CIRCULATION
- Bradycardia
- Decompensated shock +

IMMINENT ARREST

- Aggressive management of ABC including intubation
- No anticonvulsant drugs

Fever, breathlessness, AWD, CHD, asthma

APPEARANCE
- Pain responsive
- Tone ↑
- Posturing +
- DEM +

BREATHING
- Respiratory failure ±
- Relative bradypnea ±
- Respiratory distress ±

CIRCULATION
- Tachycardia/relative bradycardia
- Shock compensated/decompensated
- Liver span N/↑

HYPOXIC/HYPOPERFUSION POSTURING

- Aggressive managemant of ABC
- Specific treatment, where possible
- No anticonvulsant drugs

Fever, headache, vomiting, prolonged fits, head trauma

APPEARANCE
- Responds to pain/unresponsive
- Tone ↑
- Posturing +
- DEM ±
- Unequal pupil ±

BREATHING
- Stridor ±
- Tachypnea/bradypnea

CIRCULATION
- Relative bradycardia
- Shock ±
- BP ↑

RAISED ICT

- Manage ABC
- Early intubation by anesthetist/ICU physician
- Anticonvulsant drugs ±

Intake of medications

APPEARANCE
- Alert +
- Tone ↑↑
- Posturing +
- Oculogyric crisis ±

BREATHING
Normal

CIRCULATION
Normal

EXTRAPYRAMIDAL SYMPTOMS

No ER management

Behavioral problems

APPEARANCE
- Alert
- GTCS +

BREATHING
Normal

CIRCULATION
Normal

CONVERSION REACTION

No ER management

Developmental delay/MR

APPEARANCE
- Chronic impaired alertness
- Tone ↑
- Intermittent posturing +
- DEM +

BREATHING
Normal

CIRCULATION
Normal

DYSTONIA

No ER management

Protocol 7.2: PEMC approach: Recognition and management of convulsive and non-convulsive status epilepticus in ED

AIRWAY: Open airway, head tilt/chin lift. Jaw thrust and cervical spine stabilization if trauma is suspected oropharyngeal suction, NGT decompression, insert airway adjunct

BREATHING: Spontaneous breathing, O_2 through flow inflating ventilation device 10 L/min
Apnea: BVM with 100% O_2 10 L/min

CIRCULATION: IV Access and correct shock, if identified with 20 mL/kg NS bolus
Correct hypoglycemia with 25% dextrose 2 mL/kg

**Consider risk of cardiogenic or non-cardiogenic PE: CSE or NCSE SE > 1 hour
- H/O incessant cry/lethargy/ posturing between fever, AWD, breathlessness and GTCs
- Avoid phenytoin/FOS, consider Levetiracetam/ sodium valproate after Benzodpiazepines

Convulsive status epilepticus

GTCS > 5 min
Not regained consciousness in between 2 episodes

- Appearance: Unresponsive; Tone: Abn; Posture: Abn; GICs +
- Breathing: Airway Unstable/ apnea
- Circulation: HR: ↑; Compensated shock: ±; Liver span: N; BP: N/↑

Non-convulsive status epilepticus

Sudden onset of unresponsiveness
GTCS: ±

- Appearance: Unresponsive; Tone: Abn; Posture: Abn; Eyelid twitch: +; Nystagmus: +; Conjugate deviation: +; No GICs
- Breathing: Airway Unstable /apnea; Tachypnea
- Circulation: HR: ↑; Compensated shock: ±; Liver span: N; BP: N/↑

Hypoxia/hypoperfusion posturing**

Fever/AWD/asthma/burns/breathlessness followed by progressive LOC

- Appearance: Pain responsive; Posturing: +; Conjugate deviation; Nystagmus, Lid twitch movements; DEM: ±
- Breathing: Airway Unstable; RR: ↑↓; Grunt: ±; SCR: +; Abdominal respiration
- Circulation: HR: ↑↓; Decompensated shock: ±; Liver span: N/↑; BP: N/↓

↓

Aggressive management of hypoxia and shock
Avoid anticonvulsants (unless GTCs are noted)
Management of precipitating cause

ABC

0 min:
IV Lorazepam (0.1 mg/kg; max 5 mg) over 1 min OR
IV Midazolam (0.1 mg/kg) over 1 min OR
IV Diazepam (0.2 mg/kg; max 10 mg). Wait for 5 min after IV BZD to determine if seizure terminates
IV access not available:
Intranasal Midazolam (0.2 mg/kg) OR
Buccal Midazolam (0.2 mg/kg/d) OR
IM Midazolam (0.2 mg/kg/d) OR
Rectal Diazepam (0.2–0.5 mg/kg)

5 min: Inj. Lorazepam/Diazepam—same dosage (second dose)

20 min: Inj. Levetiracetam 20–30 mg/kg @ 5 mg/kg/min (if history of prolonged SE/SE with septic shock) if no CLD/no IEM/no bleeding:
Consider sodium valproate 20 mg/kg @ 5 mg/kg/min
Inj. phenytoin** 20 mg/kg IV loading dose; max 50 mg/min @ 1 mg/kg/min
– mix with NS; incompatible with glucose containing solutions
– monitor HR, perfusinon and BP
(or)
Inj. fosphenytoin** 30 mg/kg IV loading dose @ 3 mg/kg/min
(1.5 mg fosphenytoin = 1 mg phenytoin equivalent)

(or)
40 min: Inj. phenytoin** 10 mg/kg (second dose)
Inj. fosphenytoin** 15 mg/kg (second dose)
Inj. pyridoxine 100 mg IV start < 2 year

60 min: Plan intubation with midazolam 0.2 mg/kg bolus (max 10 mg) over 2 min
IV phenobarbitone 20 mg/kg @ 2 mg/kg/min up to a maximum of 30 mg/kg

Plan shift to PICU: Start midazolam infusion @ 1 μg/kg/min; increase every 15 min up to 33–50 μg/kg/min

ABCs stabilized fits controlled → Place child in recovery posture, shift to ward, evaluate for cause

- Intubate if SaO_2 < 92% despite effective bag-valve-mask ventilation, features of PE/cardiac dysfunction, low BP, head injury, ICP
- 10–30 mL/kg NS (shock due to idiopathic SE) > 60 mL/kg if shock due to sepsis/hypovolemia
- Avoid sodium valproate if jaundice or bleeding or suspected IEM
- Phenytoin/FOS safe if SE < 30 minute, GTCs occurs suddenly without preceding ALOC, effective prehospital care
- Continue treatment until airway stable/ET, breathing normal/apnea, HR: N, perfusion: N, liver span: N, BP: N, alert or intubated without clinical signs of SE (ambulatory EEG should be done to document there is no ongoing electrical status)

8
CHAPTER

Envenomation

Chapter Outline

- Scorpion Envenomation
- Snake Envenomation

SCORPION ENVENOMATION

PATHOPHYSIOLOGY (FIGURE 1)

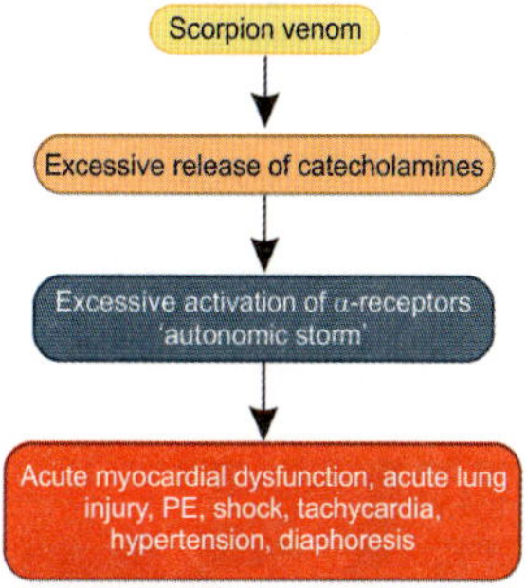

Figure 1: Pathophysiology of scorpion envenomation.

Clinical manifestations may be local or systemic. Symptoms progress to a maximum of 3-5 hours and subside within 1-2 days.

Management: Local and Systemic Effects

- Apply ice cubes to reduce pain.
- This method slows the absorption of venom by local vasoconstriction (avoid freezing the site of bite while using ice cubes).
- Prescribe paracetamol
- Avoid local infiltration of lignocaine (Inherent risk of arrhythmias is high in scorpion envenomation)
- Anti-emetics if vomiting is severe.
- Seizures are managed with benzodiazepines.
- Routine antimicrobials are not needed
- Correct dehydration.

Prazosin

Prazosin is indicated only if features of autonomic storm are identified.

- Vomiting, salivation and sweating.
- Dose: 30 micrograms/kg/dose
- Repeat every 3–4 hours till extremities become warm and dry.
- If the child vomits, the drug may be administered via the nasogastric tube.

The child is maintained in the supine posture to avoid postural hypotension.

DONTS

Never use: Lignocaine, Morphine, Steroids
Avoid infiltrating site of bite with lignocaine. It increases risk of arrhythmias.

Protocol for recognition of severity of scorpion sting and management (Figures 2A to D).

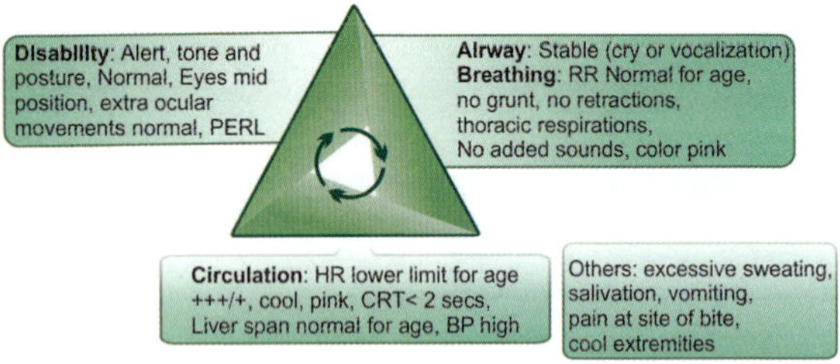

Figure 2A: Scorpion envenomation: Normal physiological status with autonomic storm.

Management: Normal physiological status with autonomic storm (Figure 2A)

- Pain relief (described above)
- T. Prazosin 0.03 mg/kg
- Avoid upright position since it can cause hypotension.

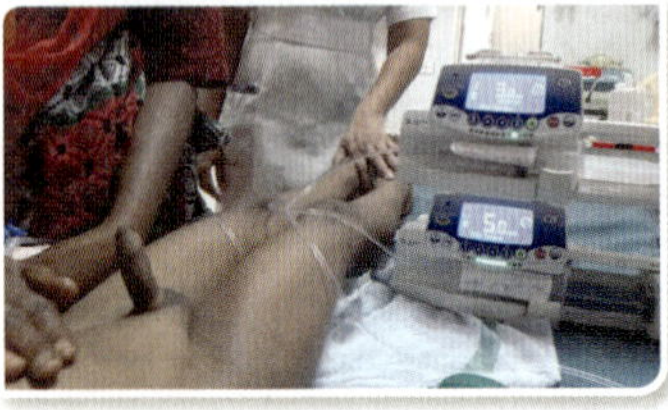

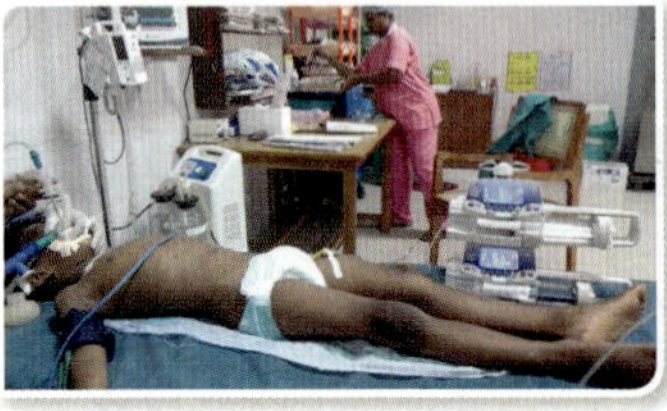

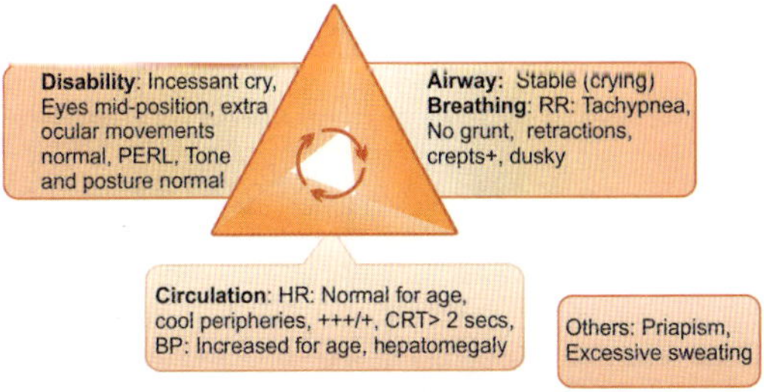

Figure 2B: Respiratory distress with cardiogenic shock due to scorpion envenomation.

Management of Cardiogenic Shock (Figure 2B)

- Oxygen via Jackson Rees circuit
- Normal saline 5–10 mL/kg aliquots (maximum 20–30 mL/kg)
- Initiate inotrope if signs of pulmonary edema are noted during fluid resuscitation.
- Dobutamine if cool shock with high BP) @ 10 mcg/kg/minute.
- Plan intubation if non-invasive ventilation fails to resolve pulmonary edema and shock
- T. Prazosin 0.03 mg/kg via NGT

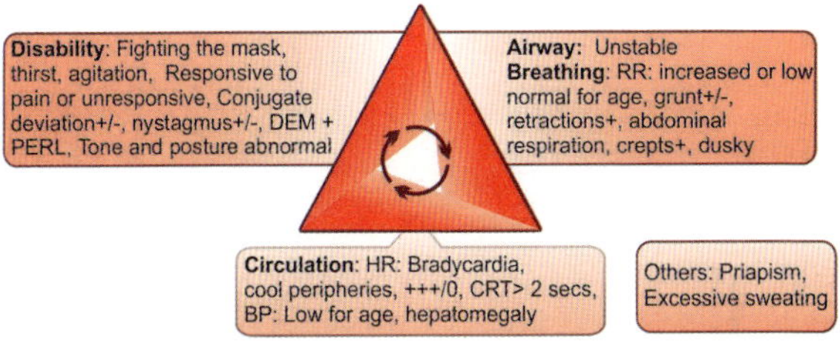

Figure 2C: Respiratory failure with hypotensive cardiogenic shock due to scorpion envenomation.

Management of hypotensive cardiogenic shock (Figure 2C)

- Oxygen via Jackson Rees circuit
- Plan early intubation (call anesthesiologist)
- Normal saline: 5–10 mL/kg boluses
- Initiate Epinephrine at 0.03–1 mcg/kg/minute
- Avoid T. Prazosin if hypotensive

Protocol 8.1: PEMC approach: Management of scorpion sting in the ED

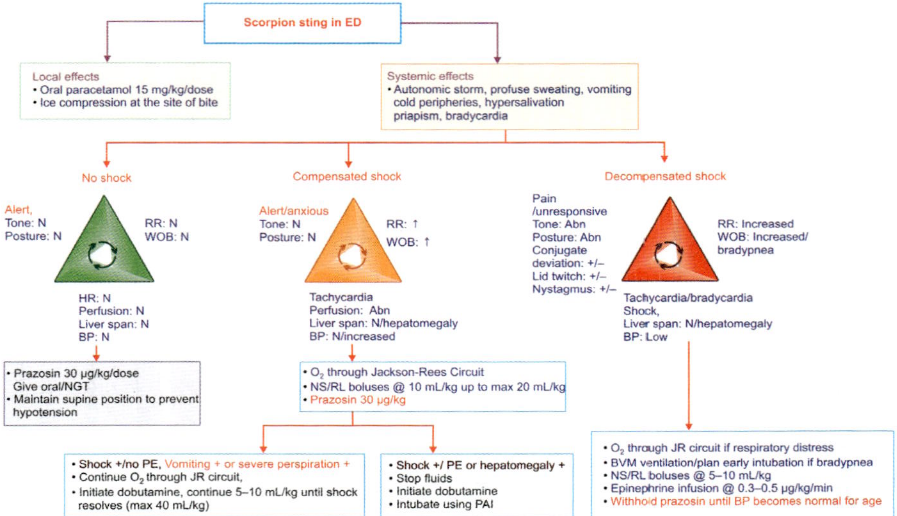

Caution:

- Risk of cardiogenic or non-cardiogenic pulmonary edema complicates shock management due to scorpion envenomation.
- During fluid therapy, monitor for airway instability, pink froth, increase or decrease in respiratory rates, grunt, retractions, abdominal respiration, fresh rales, gallop, increasing liver span, agitation, fighting the mask and drop in oxygen saturations (i.e. signs of pulmonary edema). If any one or a cluster of signs develop, stop further fluid, initiate inotropes and prepare to intubate.

SNAKE ENVENOMATION

SNAKE BITE

PATHOPHYSIOLOGY OF SNAKE VENOM

Snake venom is a complex mixture of enzymatic compounds (Phospholipases A2, D hydrolases, proteases, hyaluronidase, nucleotidase and ATPases) and non-enzymatic compounds such as neurotoxins and hemotoxins.

First Aid Treatment

"Do It RIGHT"

R: Reassure the patient

Among all victims of snake bite, non-poisonous bites account for 70%. Even if bitten by venomous snakes, only 50% of bites, lead to envenomation.

I: Immobilize, in a manner similar to that of a fractured limb.

The affected limb is splinted using bandages or cloth. Care is taken to avoid blocking blood supply. Tight ligatures are contraindicated.

GH: Get to Hospital immediately.

Traditional remedies and native medications have no proven benefit.

T: Tell the doctor of any systemic symptoms such as ptosis that manifest on the way to hospital.

DONTS

- **Do not wash the wound.**
  - Washing the wound increases the flow of venom into the system by stimulating the lymphatic system.
- **Do not apply tourniquets.**
  Increases risk of ischemia leading to necrosis of limb. Release of tourniquet, increases risk of neurotoxic blockade or embolism due to sudden release of toxin from the wound.
- **Do not incise the wound.**
  Incision increases the risk of severe bleeding.
- **Do not apply suction to the wound.**
  Suction does not reduce the amount of circulating venom. It may in fact increase envenomation and also increase the risk of necrosis at the site of bite.
- **Do not apply electric shock or cryotherapy to the wound.**
  Both measures have no benefit, but enhance the necrotic effect of the venom.
- **Avoid pressure immobilization.**
  Pressure immobilization, without appropriate training or equipment can worsen risk of necrosis.
- **Avoid, adding one vial of ASV to IV fluids prior to referral.**
  Inadequate dosing can lead to sensitization resulting in anaphylaxis and death.

Whole blood clotting time (WBCT)

Collect 1 mL of blood in a clean test tube and make note of the time of collection (Fig. 3). Failure to clot after 20 minutes is suggestive of snake envenomation.

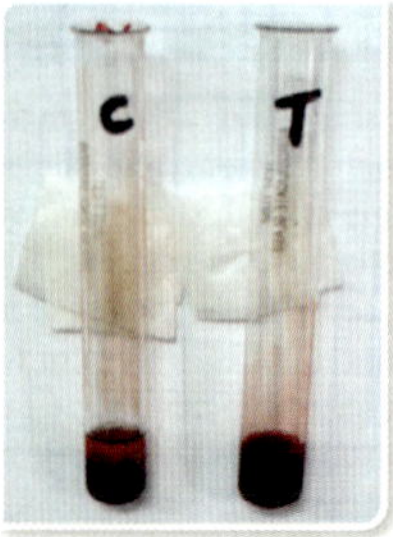

Fig. 3: WBCT after 20 minutes

APPROACH TO A VICTIM BITTEN BY A SNAKE

Determine whether the bite is by a poisonous snake.

Look for Fang Marks

- The depth of the bite varies anywhere from 1 to 8 mm. In some bite marks may not be evident.

Note Time of Bite

- Onset of poisoning may occur as early as 5 minutes or as late as 10 hours (cobra bites), 20 minutes (Viper bites).
  In regions where snake bites are common, a high index of suspicion based on symptoms and signs is needed to initiate therapy.

Local Manifestations

- Local pain, tenderness, edema, erythema or discoloration occur within 6–30 minutes.
- Tingling and numbness over the tongue, mouth and scalp are common in viper bites.
- Local bleeding, petechial and purpuric rash are common in viper bites.
- Wet gangrenous lesions and compartment syndrome are common in cobra bites.
- Regional lymphadenopathy, is a reliable sign of systemic poisoning.

Systemic Manifestation

Severe vomiting, headache, myalgia, vertigo and hypersalivation are common.

Neurological Symptoms

- Ptosis, external ophthalmoplegia, hyperacusis and weakness of muscles of palate, jaw, tongue, larynx, neck and muscles of deglutition have been noted.
- Cranial nerve involvement, drowsiness, coma and respiratory muscle paralysis are other signs of severe envenomation. (The diaphragm is the last to be affected)

Ptosis is an early sign of envenomation following bite of krait or cobra.
Hemostatic abnormalities are the hallmark of viper bites.

- Cardiotoxicity manifests as tachycardia, hypotension, myocardial infarction and cardiac arrest.
- Hypotension and shock occur due to hemorrhage, vasodilation, increased capillary permeability, acute pituitary, adrenal insufficiency (Russell's viper bites) and anaphylaxis due to ASV.
- Acute renal failure (oliguria) is a complication of viper bite-induced muscle necrosis and myoglobinuria.
- Ongoing absorption of the venom from blood (half-life of venom is between 26

and 96 hours) can lead to recurrence of symptoms.

- Frequent evaluation of the patients is essential for 3–4 days.

Indications for ASV

- Evidence of coagulopathy: WBCT >20 minutes or signs of spontaneous bleeding are noted.
- Neurotoxicity: Ptosis, inability to lift the head, diplopia, stridor, respiratory distress, neuro-paralysis or coma.
- Swelling extending:
  a. 15 cm or more within 1 hour.
  b. Swelling reaching the knee or elbow < 4 hours after bite involving the limbs.
  c. Swelling involving the whole limb within 8 hours.
  d. Extension to the trunk.
  e. Swelling causing airway compromise or shortness of breath.
  f. Compartment syndrome or major vessel entrapment.

  Painful swelling that is both progressive and severe is a definitive indication for ASV.
- Cardiovascular abnormalities: Hypotension, shock, cardiac arrhythmias.
- Persistent vomiting, abdominal pain.

> - 10 vials of ASV are diluted in 5 to 10 ml/kg of NS or 5% Dextrose or RL and infused over 1 hour at constant rate.
> - Also administer injection TT1/2 cc IM
> - Antibiotic if evidence of cellulitis.

Local wound management

a. Cleanse the wound and leave it open.
b. Mark with ink the proximal border and note the time
c. Measure the circumference
d. Elevate limb.

> *Management of envenomation is based on severity. The latter is evaluated using the rapid cardiopulmonary cerebral assessment and the pediatric assessment triangle (Figures 4A to E).*

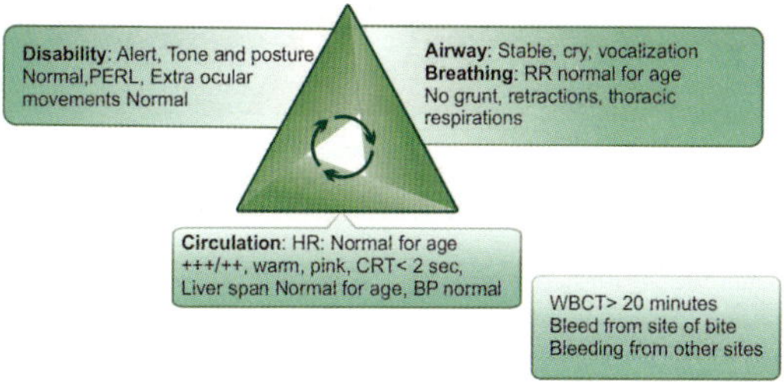

Figure 4A: Hemotoxic bite
Airway stable, **Breathing:** Normal, **Circulation:** Normal Disability: Nil

Management of Hemotoxic bite (Stable)
ASV 8-10 vials

Management of Hemotoxic Bite (Green Triangle)

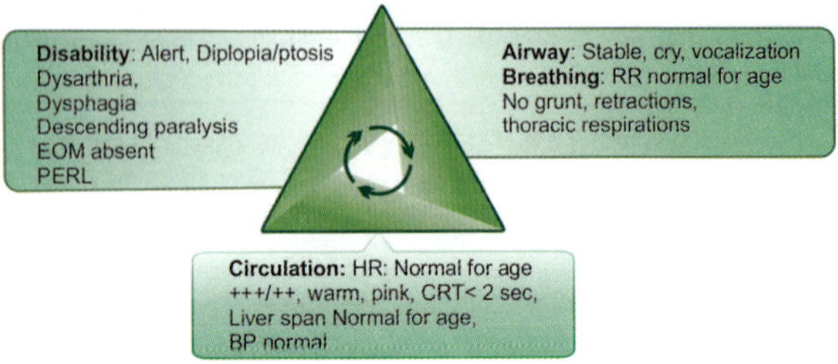

Figure 4B: Neurotoxic bite (Stable)
Airway: Stable
Breathing: Normal
Circulation: HR Normal for age, no shock, liver span normal, BP normal, Disability: No altered mental status, cranial nerve palsies

Management of Neurotoxic bite (Green triangle)

- ASV 8-10 vials (Max 20)
- Atropine 0.02 mg/kg ½ hourly with Neostigmine 50-100 mcg/kg, if no improvement repeat 2nd dose.

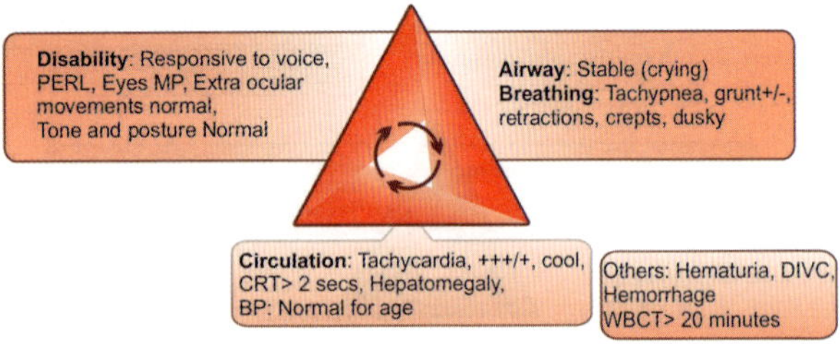

Figure 4C: Hemotoxic bite (Unstable) Respiratory distress with cardiogenic shock

Management of Hemotoxic bite (Red triangle)

- **Airway and Breathing:** O_2 via JR circuit.
- **Circulation:** 10 mL/kg NS bolus (maximum 30 mL/kg)
- Initiate dopamine at 10 mcg/kg/minute when features of pulmonary edema are un-masked.
- Plan intubation
- Plan intubation if intubation triggers are noted (*see* Protocol 8.1)

- ASV 10 vials in 100 mL of 5% GDW over 1 hour. Repeat dose every 8 hours (maximum 30 vials).
- Continue to monitor WBCT every 6 hours.
- Blood component therapy may be warranted.

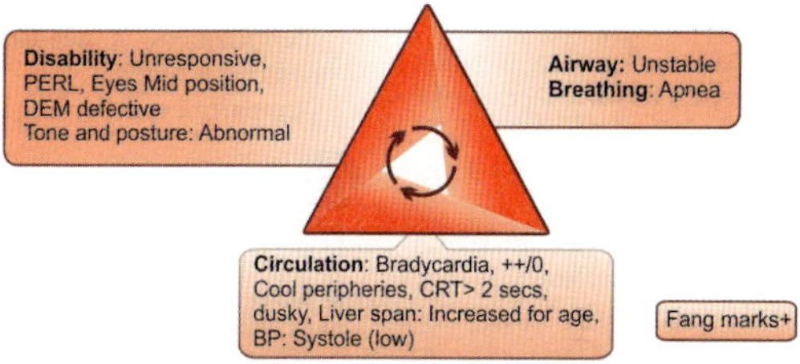

Figure 4D: Neurotoxic envenomation (Unstable): Respiratory paralysis with imminent arrest

Management of Neurotoxic Bite with Respiratory Arrest (Red triangle)

- **Airway:** Head tilt chin lift, suction oropharynx, NG decompression
- **Breathing:** Initiate BVM ventilation, (plan intubation after fluid bolus and epinephrine infusion is initiated)
- **Circulation:**
- Chest compression (15:2)
- Injection epinephrine 0.1 mL/kg (1:10,000) IV
- 10 mL/kg of NS bolus,
- Epinephrine infusion (0.5 to 1 mcg/kg/minute)
- ASV 8-10 vials in 100 mL of (5% GDW) over one hour (max 20).
- Plan Atropine 0.02-0.05 mg/kg IV + Neostigmine 0.05 to 0.1 mg/kg every ½ hour.

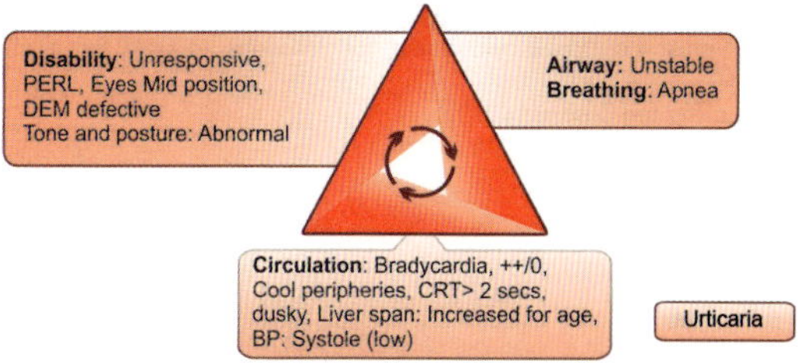

Figure 4E: Airway: Obstructed (Tongue and airway mucosa might have swelled up); **Breathing:** Respiratory distress due to bronchospasm; **Circulation:** Bradycardia with hypotensive shock **Disability:** Altered level of consciousness with or without non-convulsive status epilepticus.

Management of Anaphylactic Shock: Red triangle

- Provide oxygen via bag valve mask, plan intubation, call for anesthetist help (anticipate difficult airway)
- Adrenaline 0.01 ml/kg body weight of 1:10000 IM, repeat doses if needed every 5 minutes
- Order Epinephrine infusion 0.1-1 mg/kg/minute
- Administer NS boluses (large volume shock) until therapeutic goals of shock are resolved
- Hydrocortisone 2 mg/kg IV
- Antihistamine – Chlorphenaramine maleate 0.2 mg/kg IV
- Once patient recovers, the ASV can be re-started slowly for 10 to 15 minutes and normal rate may be resumed.

When do you call the surgeon?

- Ulcer at the site of fang marks
- Necrosis of the skin and underlying tissues
- Gangrene of the toes and fingers (debridement is needed when tissue necrosis is noted)
- Compartment syndrome

ASV 8-10 vials, 6th hourly WBCT, Fresh frozen plasma, Cryoprecipitate, fresh blood as needed, plasmapheresis if these measures fail. Monitor RFT, Urine output

Repeat WBCT every 6 hours. The liver takes 6 hours to replace the clotting factors.

KEY POINTS

1. Early and adequate dosage of anti-venom, is crucial to prevent irreversible muscle damage.
2. Avoid using smaller doses for young infants and children.
3. Administer 8–25 vials for all ages, if signs of envenomation are noted.
4. The patient must be closely monitored for reactions to ASV for a minimum of 2 hours.
5. Do not administer test dose of ASV

Protocol 8.2: PEMC approach: Management of scorpion sting in the ED

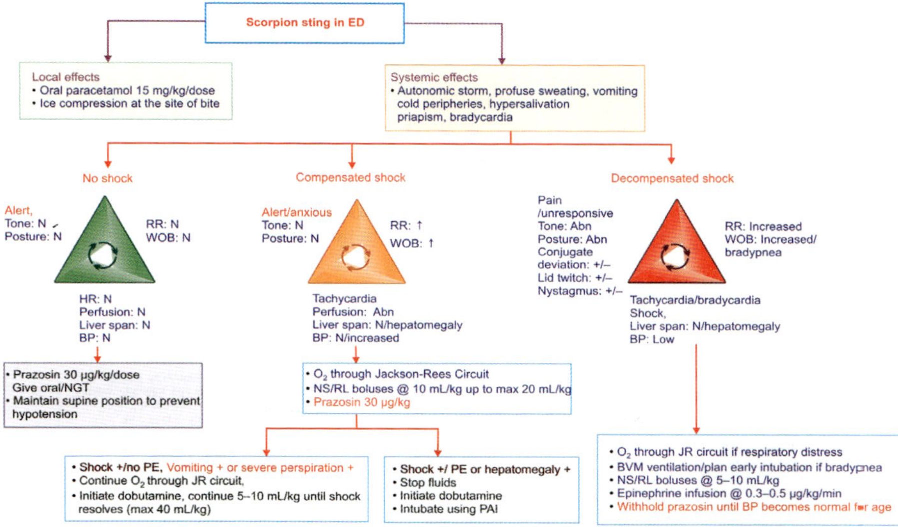

Protocol 8.3: PEMC approach to the management of snake bite in the ED

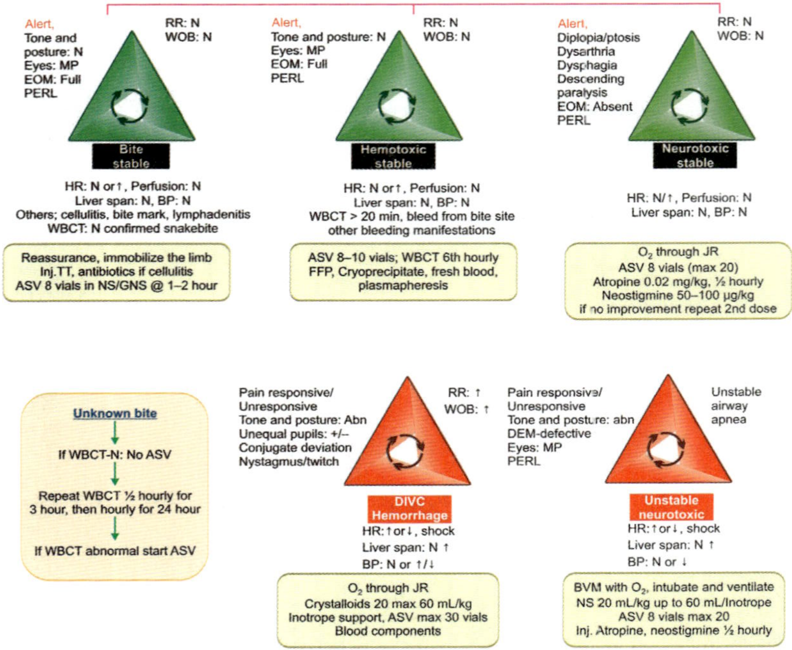

9

CHAPTER

Poisoning

In most cases, ingestion of toxic agent has minimal or no clinically important toxic effects. Rarely, the ingested amount is life-threatening resulting in death.

Early aggressive efforts to eliminate the toxin is the best guarantor for successful outcomes.

Suspect poisoning if an apparently normal child develops symptoms of organ dysfunction when an empty bottle, or tablets or spillage of house hold chemicals are noted near a child.

1. Evaluate constituents of the ingested substance.
2. Calculate its per kilogram body weight (Presume that maximum amount has been ingested by comparing the volume of liquid or number of the tablets remaining in the container).
3. Take spillage into account.

MANAGEMENT

1. Cardiopulmonary cerebral assessment and resuscitation
2. Prevention or reduction of absorption.
3. Enhancement of excretion
4. Administration of antidotes

Cardiopulmonary Cerebral Assessment and Resuscitation

- Plan early intubation, if victim presents with an unmaintainable airway or/and respiratory failure.
- Profound depression of mental status can result in airway compromise and respiratory failure (Figures 1A to C).
- Correct shock with 10–20 mL/kg isotonic fluids. Shock may occur due to vomiting and diarrhea.

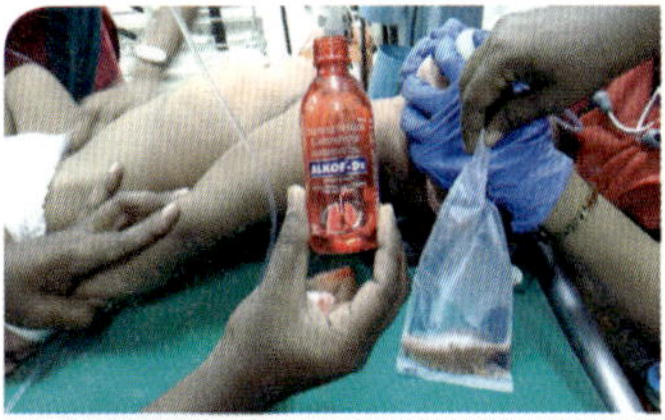

Figure 1A: Child brought unresponsive after consuming the whole bottle of cough syrup.

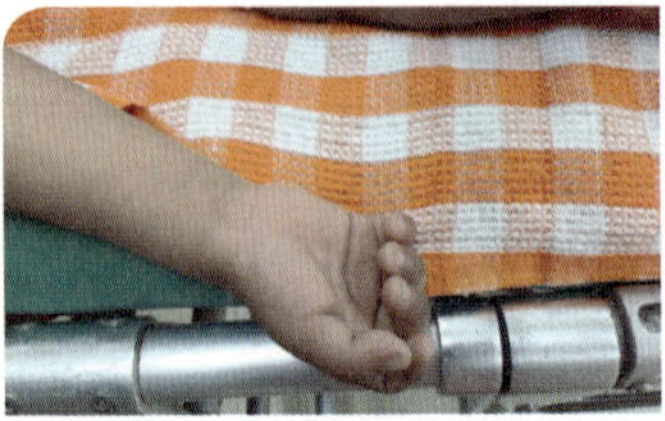

Figure 1B: Flushed palms.

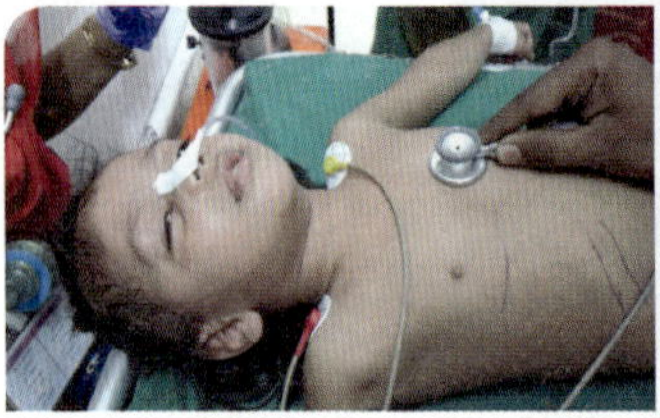

Figure 1C: Flushed facies.

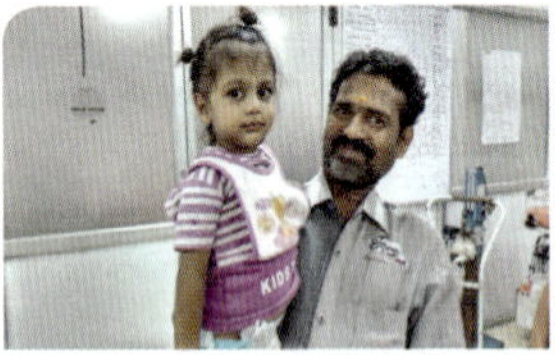

Figure 1D: Well child following intubation, ventilation, correction of cardiogenic shock and gastric decontamination.

- If cardiogenic shock is noted, initiate appropriate inotrope infusion based on blood pressure (BP) (establish euvolemia prior to starting inotrope) (Figure 2).
- Perform dextrostix and correct documented hypoglycemia with boluses of 5 mL/kg of 10% dextrose (Figure 3). Initiate intravenous fluids at maintenance rates if the victim presents with nausea and vomiting in the absence of shock.

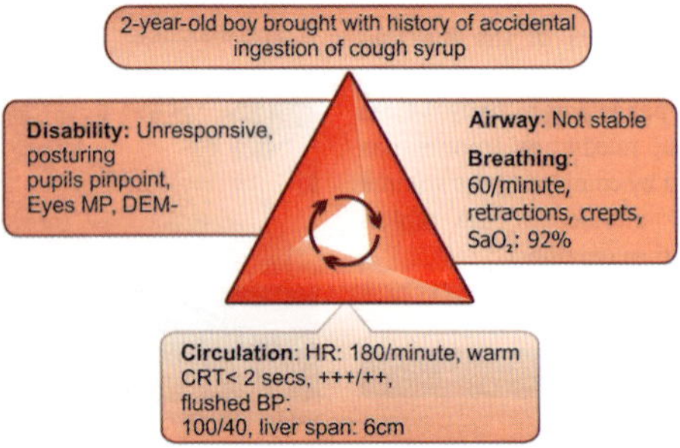

Figure 2: Airway: Not stable, Breathing: Respiratory distress circulation: Tachycardia, Normotensive vasodilatory shock, Disability: Altered level of consiousness.

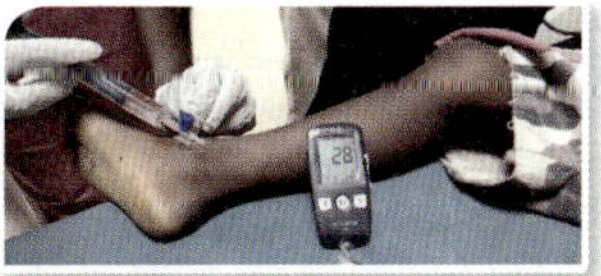

Figure 3: Correct documented hypoglycemia

- Avoid treating mild metabolic acidosis. It is encountered quite frequently, but does not require specific therapy.
- Treat convulsions using the standard protocol for status epilepticus.
- Monitor hepatic and renal function.

Arrhythmias are uncommon. If noted in a toxin victim, it will resolve when coexisting hypoxia, hypercarbia, dyselectrolytemia and acid-base abnormalities are corrected.

POISON SYNDROMES (TOXIDROMES) (TABLE 1)

Table 1: Toxidromes

Toxidromes	Associated signs	Possible toxin
Anticholinergic activity	1. Hot as a hare: Hyperthermia 2. Dry as a bone: Dry mucosa and skin 3. Red as a beet: Flushing 4. Mad as a hatter: Delirium 5. Blind as a bat: Mydriasis 6. Tachycardia 7. Urinary retention	Atropine Anti-histamine Anti-spasmodics Phenothiazines Tricyclic anti-depressants Mushroom poisoning Anti-Parkinsonian drugs
Cholinergic activity		
Muscarinic effect	1. Salivation 2. Lacrimation 3. Urination 4. Defecation 5. Gastrointestinal cramping 6. Emesis 7. Miosis	Organophosphorus toxins (insecticides) (Figure 5)
Nicotinic effect		
Stimulation followed by paralysis of preganglionic and somatic nerve fibers, excessive cholinergic stimulation of the motor end-plate	Fasciculations, weakness, paralysis	Organophosphorus poisons

Contd...

Contd...

Toxidromes	Associated signs	Possible toxin
Sympathetic nervous system activity	Fever, flushing, tachycardia, hypertension, miosis, sweating	Cough and decongestants, theophylline
Methemoglobinemia	Cyanosis resistant to oxygen	Aniline dyes, nitrates, benzocaine, phenacetin, nitrobenzene, chlorates
Acute ataxia and nystagmus		Antihistamines, alcohol, anticonvulsants, bromides, organic solvents
Metabolic acidosis	Effortless tachypnea	Ethanol, carbon monoxide, iron, diabetic medications, salicylates, tricyclic antidepressants
Renal failure Oliguria, anuria, hematuria, myoglobinuria Carbon tetrachloride, ethylene glycol, methanol, mushrooms, oxalates		

Toxins can result in a cluster of signs, which help to recognize the specific agent.

Perform a complete neurological assessment, while resuscitation is in progress. It could reveal clues which point towards

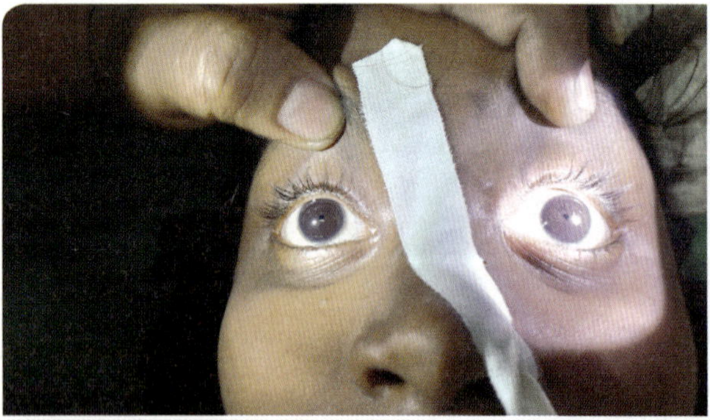

Figure 4: Note the pin -point pupils of organo phosphorous poisoning.

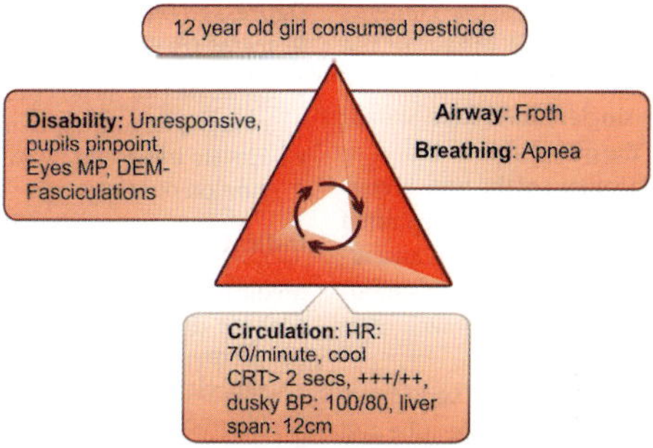

Figure 5: A: Froth **B:** Apnea **C:** Bradycardia, shock (normotensive), ALOC with pin point pupils and fasciculations. This child, received bag valve mask ventilation, one bolus of 20 ml/kg. She received Injection Atropine 0.05 mg/kg. The dose was doubled every 5 minutes until hypoxia, bradycardia reverted and secretions dried up.

the specific toxin especially when history is unavailable (Figure 4).

Reduction of Absorption

- Routine induction of emesis is not recommended in the management of toxin ingestion.

> *Gastric lavage should not be employed routinely*

- Unless intubated, gastric lavage is contraindicated in children whose airway protective reflexes are lost.
- Gastric lavage is contraindicated if a hydrocarbon with high aspiration potential has been ingested.
- Gastric lavage is also contraindicated if a corrosive substance has been ingested.
- Gastric lavage can be considered when a potentially life-threatening amount of a poison has been ingested.

Patients, who are more likely to benefit from aggressive gastrointestinal decon-tamination:

- Obtunded patients presenting very soon after ingestion.
- Ingestion of a life-threatening or massive amount.
- Drugs that could delay gastric emptying.
- Ingestion of sustained release tablets.

Method

1. Competence of the gag reflex should first be confirmed.

- Once properly restrained, the child should be placed in a left lateral decubitus (Trendelenburg position) in order to limit the movement of the gastric contents into the duodenum and minimize the risk of aspiration.

- A large bore, single lumen tube should be placed via the oro-gastric route.
- The proper placement of the tube is confirmed by the spontaneous or aspirated return of gastric contents or by auscultation of insufflated air when a stethoscope is placed over the stomach after placement of the tube.
- NS in aliquots of 10–15 mL/kg of body weight are instilled through the tube and then aspirated. This process is continued until the aspirated contents are clear. Volumes as large as several liters may be necessary to produce a clear aspirate.

Activated Charcoal

- Activated charcoal should be administered within 1 hour of ingestion of toxin.
- Recommended dose is 1 g/kg body weight

Method of Administration

Normal Mental Status

- Mix activated charcoal in fruit juice or bottled drinks as a slurry.
- Additives, such as bottled drinks or fruit juices, make charcoal more palatable without reducing its efficacy.
- Young children will not voluntarily drink activated charcoal quickly enough for it to work optimally.
- Hence, the nasogastric tube is introduced in young children in order to ensure prompt administration.

Depressed Mental Status or Respiratory Failure

- Intubate (for airway protection) and use nasogastric tube for administration.
- Elevate head-end by 45° during administration of AC.

Indications for Activated Charcoal

Medications that are well bound by charcoal are drugs that undergo enterohepatic or enteroenteric circulation such as:

1. Salicylates
2. Phenobarbital
3. Carbamazepine
4. Digoxin
5. Theophylline

Substances which are not adsorbed by activated charcoal are remembered by the mnemonic PHAILS:

P : Pesticides
H : Hydrocarbons
A : Acids, alkalis, alcohols
I : Iron
L : Lithium
S : Solvents

Catharsis

Commonly used osmotic agents are magnesium citrate and sorbitol. These agents promote retention of colonic fluid and stimulate gastrointestinal motility.

Currently Cathartic Agents are Contraindicated

The risk of hypernatremic dehydration and cardiovascular collapse is high with sorbitol, while hypermagnesemia is a hazard in children with renal disease.

Whole Bowel Irrigation (WBI)

In this procedure, large volumes of solution are administered enterally until the rectal effluent is clear. Polyethylene glycol-electrolyte (PEGLEC) lavage solution has been formulated to prevent extensive absorption or secretion of fluid across the gastrointestinal mucosa.

- Elevate head-end of bed to at least 45° to prevent aspiration.
- Discontinue the infusion for 30 minutes, if emesis occurs and restart at half the previous rate.
- Increase the rate as tolerated
- Administer Metoclopramide (antiemetic), since it increases GI motility.
- Provide a bedside commode for patients who are awake.

Whole bowel irrigation is safe in children, volumes as large as 44 L have been administered without ill effects. Typical rates of administration are 500–1,000 mL/h, orally or by nasogastric tube. The adverse effects associated with this procedure consist of vomiting, abdominal cramps and bloating.

Urine Alkalinization

Urine alkalinization is a treatment regimen that increases elimination of poison by the administration of intravenous sodium bicarbonate to produce urine with a pH of 7.5. The term 'urine alkalinization' emphasizes that urine pH manipulation rather than a diuresis as the prime objective of treatment.

- Consider urine alkalinization as first-line treatment for patients who have moderately severe salicylate poisoning.
- Urine alkalinization cannot be recommended as first-line treatment in cases of phenobarbital poisoning as multiple-dose-activated charcoal is superior.
- Common house hold items are often ingested. These items have low toxicity (Table 3).

Another common source of toxins include medications. Occasionally, even one pill can kill. The most common "two pills can kill" list includes, sodium channel blockers such as chloroquine, dextropropoxyphene, propranolol, tricyclic antidepressants, calcium channel blockers (CCBs), diphenoxylate/atropine, dextropropoxyphene, beta-blockers, sulfonylureas, and theophylline slow release.

Toxic effects occurring within a few hours:

- Chloroquine: Rapid onset of coma, seizures, hypotensive shock.
- Dextropropoxyphene: VT
- Propranolol: Coma, seizures, ventricular dysrhythmias, hypoglycemia
- Tricyclic antidepressants: Coma, seizures, ventricular tachycardia, hypotension.

Toxic effects occurring between 8–12 hours:

- Hypoglycemia, occurring within the first 8 hours point toward sulfonylurea toxicity.
- Verapamil, diltiazem: Late onset conduction defects, bradycardia, hypotension and refractory shock;
- Opioids: Coma, respiratory depression, pinpoint pupils;
- Theophylline sustained-release: Vomiting, seizures, SVT.

Table 2: Dos and don'ts for toxins and tablet poisoning

Toxins							
Poison	**Toxic dose**	**Dos**	**Don'ts**	**Elimination**	**Antidote**	**Route of adminis-tration**	**Dose and administration**
Paracetamol acetaminophen (APAP)	Single dose—200 mg/kg Consecutive days— > 90 mg/kg/day (supra-therapeutic doses)	• Symptomatic: Treat immediately • Asymptomatic and AST raised: Treat immediately • APAP is >10 µg/mL, treat even though asymptomatic and AST is normal • Oral antidote is better than IV	Symptomatic: Do not wait for lab results Ingestion more than 24 hours ago APAP, not useful Do not use Rumack Matthew nomogram for supra-therapeutic doses or when ingestion was more than 24 hours ago	Activated charcoal within 1–2 hrs of ingestion	N-Acetyl Cysteine	Oral IV	140 mg/kg loading, followed by 70 mg/kg q4h 150 mg/kg over 1 hr, followed by 50 mg/kg over 4 hrs, followed by 100 mg/kg over 16 hrs
Iron	> 40 mg/kg: Refer for urgent medical evaluation	• Serum levels after 4–6 hrs of ingestion • Treat if > 500 µg/dl Or • Moderate to severe symptoms	• Do not use activated charcoal • Caution when Desferroxamine is infused for prolonged duration. It can cause pulmonary toxicity and Yersinia sepsis	Whole bowel irrigation	Deferoxamine	IV infusion	Infusion @ 5–15 mg/kg/hr (max: 6 g/24 hrs)

Contd...

Contd...

Toxins

Poison	Toxic dose	Dos	Don'ts	Elimination	Antidote	Route of administration	Dose and administration
Digoxin	Plasma digoxin levels 0.5–2.0 ng/ml (therapeutic concentration) > 2 ng/ml: Toxic > 6 ng/ml: Potentially fatal	• Take blood for serum levels after 6 hours of ingestion • Fab fragments indicated if 1. life-threatening dysrhythmias 2. K+ value >5–5.5 mEq/L 3. Serum digoxin > 15 ng/mL at any time or > 10 ng/mL after ingestion 4. Total ingestion > 4 mg 5. Hypotension or cardiovascular instability 6. Altered mental status 7. Renal failure (K >5.5 mEq/L predicts poor outcome)	Avoid co-administration of medications that increase serum digoxin levels, etc. • Macrolides, erythromycin, clarithromycin, • Spirinolactone, • Verapamil, • Amiodarone, • Itraconazole	Activated charcoal	Digoxin-specific Fab antibodies (Digibind; DigiFab)	Intravenous	One vial binds 0.6 mg of digitalis glycoside #vials = digitalis level × weight in kg/100

Contd...

Contd...

Toxins							
Poison	**Toxic dose**	**Dos**	**Don'ts**	**Elimination**	**Antidote**	**Route of administration**	**Dose and administration**
Organo-phosphorous compounds	Even small amount	• Decontamination • Remove all exposed clothing • Measure RBC cholinesterase and pseudo-cholinesterase levels	• Activated charcoal not useful • Pralidoxime not necessary for carbamate poisoning • Avoid succinylcholine for RSI	• Decontamination • Washing all exposed parts with soap and water • Gastric lavage can be tried if brought within 1 hour and large quantity had been ingested	Atropine Pralidoxime (2–PAM)	IV/ET IV/IM	0.05–0.1 mg/kg repeated every 5–10 min as needed 25–50 mg/kg over 5–10 min (max: 200 mg/min); can be repeated after 1–2 hr, then q10–12 hr as needed
Anticholinergic agents	Lethal dose 4 mg	• > 102° F: External cooling • Maintain hydration • Benzodiazepines for agitation or seizures		• Activated charcoal 1 g/kg • Gastric lavage if large quantity has been ingested and child brought within 1 hour	Physostigmine	IV/IM	0.02 mg/kg over 5 min; may be repeated ever 5–10 min to max 2 mg
Opioids	Fatal dose: Oral > 0.3 g Parenteral > 0.1 g	• Minimum hospitalization for 24 hours		• Gastric lavage can be tried if brought	Naloxone	IV	0.01–0.1 mg/kg; adolescents/adults: 0.04–2

Contd...

Contd...

Toxins

Poison	Toxic dose	Dos	Don'ts	Elimination	Antidote	Route of adminis-tration	Dose and administra-tion
		• ECG monitoring • Methadone indicated if QTc prolongation is noted • Magnesium infusion is prepared if Torsades de pointes is noted		within 1 hour and large quantity had been ingested			mg, repeated as needed may be given continuous infusion
Dapsone	Toxic dose is close to therapeutic dose Even 100 mg is toxic	• Monitor methemoglobin levels • Since the half-life is long, children can be discharged with ascorbic acid • Correct associated acidosis • Exchange transfusion can be tried in some situations		Gastric lavage	Methylene blue, 1% solution	IV	0.1–0.2 mL/kg (1–2 mg/kg) over 5–10 min; can be repeated every 30–60 min
Methemoglobinemia					Methylene blue, 1% solution	IV	0.1–0.2 mL/kg (1–2 mg/kg) over 5–10 min; can be repeated every 30–60 min

Contd...

Contd...

Toxins

Poison	Toxic dose	Dos	Don'ts	Elimination	Antidote	Route of administration	Dose and administration
Benzodiazepines		Bag valve mask ventilation for respiratory insufficiency	Do not exceed cumulative dose of 5 mg If more than 5 mg of flumazenil is needed, the cause of sedation is not BZD	Gastric lavage if ingested within 1 hour	Flumazenil	IV	0.002–0.02 mg/kg over 30 sec; if response is inadequate—repeat as needed Max 5 mg
Methanol ethylene glycol	Toxic dose 10–30 mL 100 mg/kg Even lower dose can cause blindness Lethal above 60–240 mL (340 mg/kg) 30 mL of 100% methanol considered fatal	If methanol blood levels are not readily available, osmolar gap estimation may be used as a surrogate marker Fomepizole is indicated if: 1. Ethylene glycol or methanol level >20 mg/dL 2. History of potentially toxic ingestion (e.g., any intentional overdose) 3. History of ingestion with evidence of acidosis	Gastric decontamination not of much value due to rapid absorption of compounds Normal osmolar gap does not rule out ingestion of any alcohol		Fomepizole	IV	15 mg/kg loading; 10 mg/kg every 12 hrs × 4 doses; 15 mg/kg every 12 hrs until EG level is < 20 mg/dL

Contd...

Contd...

Toxins

Poison	Toxic dose	Dos	Don'ts	Elimination	Antidote	Route of administration	Dose and administration
		Indications for dialysis: 1. Methanol level of > 50 mg/dL 2. Acidosis 3. Severe electrolyte disturbances 4. Renal failure Therapy should be continued until ethylene glycol and methanol levels are < 20 mg/dL					
Carbon monoxide		Hyperbaric oxygen—HBO for severely poisoned	Do not mistake for flu or food poisoning	Inhalation of oxygen	Oxygen	Inhalational	100% FiO_2 via non–rebreather mask (or ET if intubated)
		Indications: Syncope, coma, seizure, altered mental status, acute coronary syndrome, HbCO level > 25%, abnormal cerebellar examination					

Tablet poisoning

Poison	Toxic dose	Dos	Don'ts	Elimination	Antidote	Route of administration	Dose and administration
Tricyclic antidepressant	Even 1 or 2 pills 10–20 mg/kg	Stabilize ABCD: • Obtain ECG as soon as possible • QRS duration of >100 msec identifies patients who are at risk for seizures and cardiac arrhythmias.	• Do not discharge prematurely • Minimum observation for 6 hours • Physostigmine relatively contraindicated	• Gastric lavage using activated charcoal	Sodium bicarbonate	IV	Bolus 1–2 mEq/kg; repeat bolus as needed to keep QRS < 110 msec
		• R wave in lead aVR of ≥ 3 mm independent predictor of toxicity Indications for sodium bicarbonate: 1. QRS duration ≥ 110 msec 2. ventricular dysrhythmias 3. Hypotension 4. 3% NS and lipid emulsion in refractory cases					
Isoniazid	20 mg/kg	• Order ABG to document metabolic acidosis • Correct acidosis if identified • Treat seizures (Refer to chapter on GTCs) • CBG: Look for hyperglycemia • Forced diuresis or hemodialysis may be warranted	Phenytoin contraindicated for INH-induced seizures	Gastric lavage	Pyridoxine	IV	Empirical dosing: 70 mg/kg (max dose = 5 g) If ingested dose is known: 1 gm for every gram of INH

Contd...

Contd...

Tablet poisoning

Poison	Toxic dose	Dos	Don'ts	Elimination	Antidote	Route of administration	Dose and administration
Beta blocker	One pill can kill Propranolol most toxic	• Supportive care • QRS widening treat with sodium bicarbonate • Seizures: Treat with BZD • Sustained release and highly lipid-soluble drugs: Observe for longer period	Not necessary to measure serum levels of beta blockers	Gastro-intestinal decontamination	Glucagon	IV	0.15 mg/kg bolus followed by infusion of 0.05–0.15 mg/kg/hr
Calcium channel blocker	Even one pill can kill Diltaizem and verapamil most dangerous in overdose	• Measure BP, • Blood glucose • At least 24 hours of observation before discharge	Profound hypotension is associated with alertness	Activated charcoal Whole bowel irrigation for sustained release product	• Insulin • Calcium salts	IV IV	1 unit/kg bolus followed by infusion of 0.5–1 unit/kg/hr Dose depends on the specific calcium salt
Rodenticide zinc phosphide	Fatal dose 5 g	• Observe for garlic odor of zinc phosphide • Gastric lavage followed by saline catharsis • Monitor hepatic and renal functions • Frequent cardiopulmonary assessment—phosphine gas is a potent respiratory toxin and can cause arrhythmias and myocarditis • Follow-up for strictures	Oil-based catharsis contraindicated	Gastric lavage with a 1 : 1000 solution of potassium permanganate			
Anticoagulant					Vitamin K		

Contd...

Contd...

Toxin poison							
Poison	**Toxic dose**	**Dos**	**Don'ts**	**Elimination**	**Antidote**	**Route of adminis-tration**	**Dose and administra-tion**
Button battery	• > 12 mm • < 12mm in < 12 years • Any size symp-tomatic	NPO until X-ray is taken to confirm position of battery in oesophagus Negative pole has a smaller diameter Expect more complications in the negative pole of the battery	• Do not induce vomiting • Do not push battery from oesophagus into stomach. This can increase risk of perforation of the oesopha-gus	If button battery has passed beyond the oesophagus spontaneously, allow for spontaneous expulsion. Inspect stools for battery	No specific antidote		
		Plan for immediate removal of battery lodged in the oesophagus (can cause serious burns within 2 hours)	• Avoid Ipecac, Laxatives, PEG-LEG solution	Endoscopic removal if: 1. Magnet is ingested 2. Symptomatic related to battery 3. Large battery ≥ 15 mm ingested by a child < 6 yrs that remains in stomach for 4 days or longer			
Corrosive acids	Sulphuric acid 3–7 mL Nitric acid 5–10 mL Hydrochloric acid- 5–15 mL	Manage ABC Broad spectrum antibiotic—3rd generation cepha-losporins No role for Corti-costeroids	Gastric lavage contraindicated Avoid barium swallow				

Contd...

Contd...

Toxin poison

Poison	Toxic dose	Dos	Don'ts	Elimination	Antidote	Route of adminis-tration	Dose and adminis-tration
Phenol	Fatal dose: 10 to 15 g or 20 drops of pure phenol	Surgery for sequalae Gastric lavage done immediately only for carbolic acid					
		in corrosive acids by passing a soft stomach tube Renal function tests Look for urine color—carboluria					
Kerosene	Fatal dose 30 mL	CPAP for respiratory distress Correct shock if identified (10–20 mL of NS) Chest x-ray after 6 hours Observation for at least 24 hrs	Emesis, gastric lavage, activated charcoal is contraindicated Routine prophylaxis with antibiotics is not necessary				
Salicy-lates	Acute toxic dose— > 150 mg/kg Significant toxicity— > 300 mg/kg Fatal dose > 500 mg/kg Even 1 teaspoon 5 g in 5 mL—severe toxicity	• Order ABG—primary respiratory alkalosis and primary anion gap metabolic acidosis • Order acetaminophen level • Order CXR—noncardiogenic pulmonary edema	• For chronic exposure, gastric decontamination is not useful • Avoid hypokalemia— as it impairs alkalinization	• Gastric decontamination with activated charcoal • Urinary alkalinization	• Sodium bicarbonate	IV	1–2 mEq/kg bolus followed by continuous infusion

Contd...

Contd...

Toxin							
Poison	**Toxic dose**	**Dos**	**Don'ts**	**Elimination**	**Antidote**	**Route of adminis-tration**	**Dose and administration**
		• Suspect bezoar formation—if salicylate concentration continues to rise after many hours of inges-tion despite treatment • Therapeutic levels are 10–20 mg/dL Levels > 30 mg/dL warrant treatment Severe toxicity—dialysis					
Cyanide	0.15 mg of hydro-cyanic acid per liter of air for a period of 20–30 min 100–200mg of cya-nide of potash Sixty drops of crude oil of bitter almond	Observe odor of bitter almonds Manage respira-tory paralysis—most common cause of death		Removal from source of exposure and high concentration of oxygen	Cyanide kit: Amyl nitrate Sodium nitrate Sodium thiosu fate		1 crushable ampule; inhale 30 sec of each min 0.33 mL/kg of 3% solution if blood level is not known; otherwise, based on tables with product

Contd...

Contd...

Toxin							
Poison	Toxic dose	Dos	Don'ts	Elimination	Antidote	Route of adminis-tration	Dose and administration
					Hydroxo-cobalamin (Cyanokit) preferred		1.6 mL/kg of 25% solution; may be repeated every 30–60 min to max of 50 mL 70 mg/kg (adults: 5 g) given over 15 min
Sulphonylureas oral hypogly-cemics	One tablet can be dangerous	Monitor for euglycemia for at least 8 hours	Repeated IV dextrose boluses and continuous dextrose infusions should be avoided as it stimulates further insulin release Prophylactic IV dex-trose infusions are not recommended -they can mask the symptoms of toxic-ity and stimulate further insulin secretion		Octreotide and dextrose	IV/SC	1–2 µg/kg/dose every 6–8 hr Adults 50–100 µg
Metformin		Hemodialysis for metformin associated lactic acidosis		Hemodialysis			

Contd...

Contd...

Toxin							
Poison	**Toxic dose**	**Dos**	**Don'ts**	**Elimination**	**Antidote**	**Route of adminis-tration**	**Dose and administration**
Lead	Blood lead levels (BLL) > 100 µg (Life-threatening) Adverse effects for chronic exposure- > 5 µg/dL	Chelation-indicated when: BLL > 45 µg/dL • 44–70 µg/dL—single drug DMSA • > 70 µg/Dl with encephalopathy: 2 drugs are used CaNa2EDTA and BAL • Without encephalopathy—CaNa2EDTA and BAL/DMSA • Repeat chelation if BLL rebounds > 45 µg/dl after a gap of 3 days • Manage PICA • Dietary counselling		Early screening reduces need for chelation	BAL dimercaprol	Deep IM	3–5 mg/kg/dose every 4 hr, for the 1st day; subsequent dosing depends on the toxin
					• Calcium disodium EDTA	IV	35–50 mg/kg/day for 5 days; continuous infusion or 2 divided doses/day
					• Dimercaptosuccinic acid (succimer, DMSA, Chemet)	Per oral	10 mg/kg/dose every 8 h for 5 days, then 10 mg/kg every 12 h for 14 days

Table 3: Common household things of low toxicity

No treatment required	
Bar soap	Lipstick
Dry cells	Newspaper
Candles	Pencil
Chalk	Shampoo
Clay (Modelling)	Shaving cream and lotions
Crayons	Shoe polish
Dehumidifying packets	Striking surface of matches
Detergents	Sweetening agents
Hand lotion and creams	Thermometer
Ink	Tooth paste
Removal necessary only if large amounts ingested	
After shave lotion	Body conditioners
Colognes	Deodorants
Fabric softeners	Hair dyes
Hair tonic	Marker ink
Matchstic >20	Oral contraceptive
Perfumes	Toilet water

KEY POINTS

1. Energetic emergency care and elimination of toxin is key to survival in the poisoned victim.
2. Emesis has been replaced by activated charcoal and whole bowel irrigation.
3. Gastric lavage should not be performed routinely in all children with toxin ingestion.
4. Consider poisoning in an apparently normal child with profound fall in mental status.
5. Avoid performing gastric lavage for minimal ingestion.
6. Use activated charcoal or whole bowel irrigation for appropriate toxins.

10

CHAPTER

Trauma and Burns

Chapter Outline

- Trauma
- Burns

PRIMARY SURVEY

Airway with Cervical Spine Protection

- Open the airway using the jaw thrust maneuver (Figure 1A).
- Suction oropharyngeal secretions.
- Jaw thrust can also provided by facing the victim (Figure 1B).

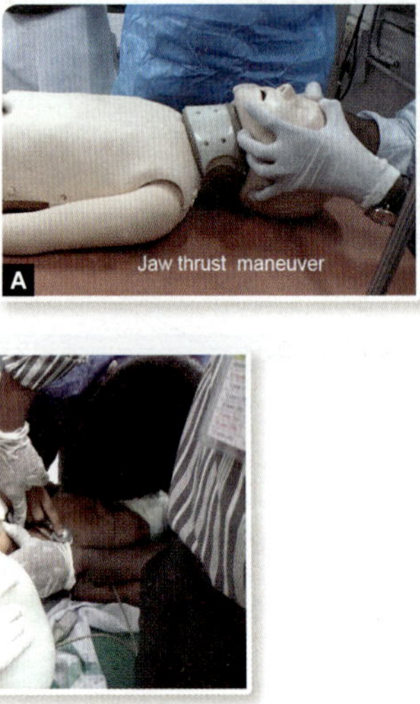

Figures 1A and B: (A) Jaw thrust maneuver; (B) Open airway, facing the victim.

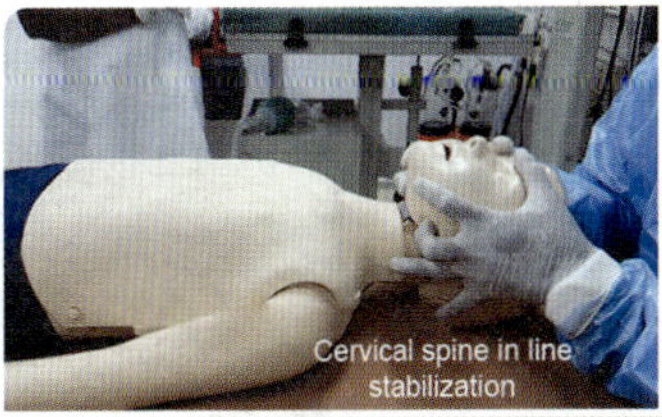

Figure 2: In-line cervical immobilization.

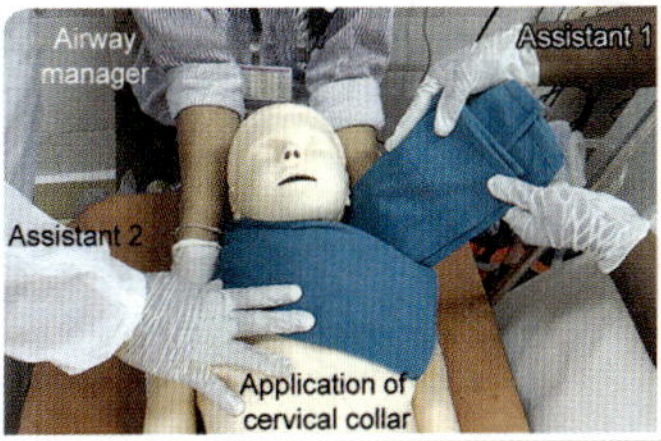

Figure 4: Application of improvised cervical collar using a thick towel. Airway manager, stabilizes the spine manually. Two assistants are needed to fix the towel. Note: The airway manager, manually stabilizes the spine while, two assistants are helping to fix the towel.

Introduce orogastric tube if altered mental status is noted or abdominal trauma is suspected. Avoid nasogastric tube.

C-spine, is presumed injured in all trauma victims who have sustained significant injuries or fall. Failure to provide C-spine immobilization can precipitate quadriplegia (Figures 2 to 6).

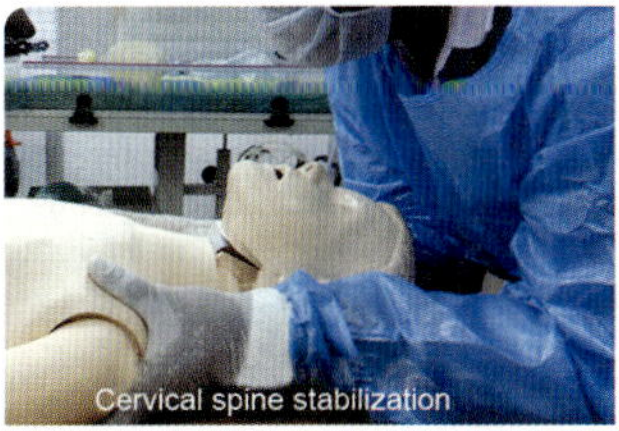

Figure 3: Cervical stabilization can also be performed by holding the head whilst concurrently fixing both shoulders.

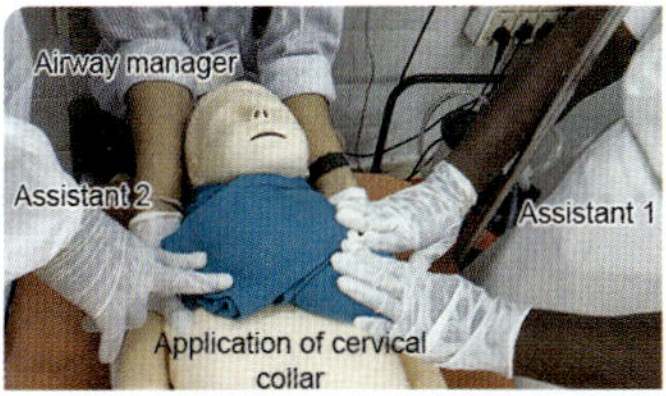

Figure 5: The towel is crossed anteriorly. The towel is fixed such that it prevents movements of the neck during transfer or imaging.

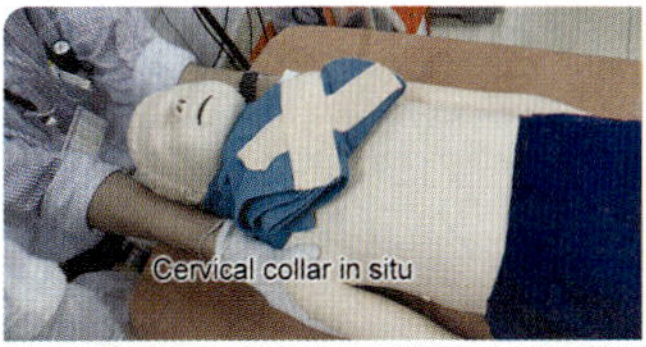

Figure 6: Dynaplast is used to fix the towel in position. Note, that the airway manager is still manually stabilizing the neck and spine.

Cervical spine stabilization in the neutral position should be maintained not only throughout resuscitation but also during transport for imaging. These precautions are taken until bony or ligamentous injuries have been excluded. If immobilization device is not available, use rolled towels (thick) or sand bags secured against the side of the neck.

The larger head in infants and children less than 4 years results in flexion of the neck when placed supine on flat surfaces.

- Use a spinal board with hollow beneath the head.
- Place folded towel under the shoulders.

Children presenting with head trauma, neck pain or neurological deficit are considered at greater risk of cervical cord injury.

Plan early intubation (Call for anesthetist) if the victim is:

- Responsive to pain or unresponsive.
- Craniofacial injuries.
- Inhalational injuries due to burns.
  - Talking or crying suggests that the airway is patent.

Breathing

- Provide oxygen using the non-rebreathing mask if spontaneously breathing.
- Check respiratory rate, work of breathing, air-entry.
- If not breathing adequately, initiate bag-valve-mask ventilation and plan early intubation.

In the absence of obvious external injury or cervical cord transection, if the child has unexplained hypotensive shock despite initial fluid bolus, suspect tension pneumothorax. Perform needle thoracocentesis to rule out this life-threatening emergency.

Do not delay needle thoracocentesis in order to take a chest X-ray if tension pneumothorax is suspected.

Circulation

- If shock is noted, 20 mL/kg of normal saline is administered up to a maximum of 50 mL/kg, if shock persists, plan blood transfusion.
- Blood is collected for grouping and cross-matching.

Fresh whole blood preferable if hypotensive and intra-abdominal injury is suspected. Bolus must be administered cautiously to avoid dislodging clots (permissive hypotension).

- Apply direct pressure if obvious bleeding is noted.
- Splint bones if obviously fractured.
- Wrap and splint pelvis to reduce bleeding into pelvic or retroperitoneal space due to pelvic fractures.

Rapid shift to operating room is planned if hypotension is noted.

Disability

- Mental status is evaluated in the AVPU scale.
- Check pupils for reaction and size along with eye position and movements for non-convulsive status epilepticus in unresponsive children.
- Avoid performing dolls eye maneuver in unresponsive victim. Neck movements can precipitate quadriplegia if the cervical cord is injured.
- Evaluate for spontaneous movement. Note presence of posturing or seizure activity.
- Assess for pain and sensation.
- Look for obvious limb deformities.

Exposure

- Remove clothing and diaper for complete secondary survey.
- Burns are calculated using the patient's palmar surface as 1%.
- If burns are noted, the affected surface is covered by moist saline dressing.

SECONDARY SURVEY

Secondary survey is a rapid evaluation for injuries prior to transfer for definitive care. During secondary survey, remember to continue to provide jaw thrust while concurrently, manually stabilizing the neck and spine.

Head and Skull (Figure 7)

- Scalp lacerations are a major cause of loss of blood, resulting in shock in young children. Saline irrigation, debridement

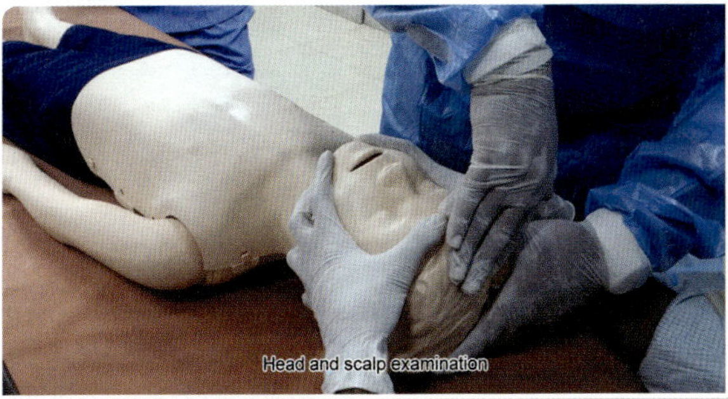

Figure 7: Examination of head and scalp while still maintaining the jaw thrust maneuver.

and suturing should be performed at the earliest.

- Bulging anterior fontanel suggests intracranial injury.
- Depressed fontanel is a sign of hypovolemia.

Maxillofacial and Intraoral Trauma (Figure 8)

- Check for nasal and oral patency. Edema could develop during fluid resuscitation in children presenting with cranio-facial trauma.
- Intubate early for significant maxillofacial trauma.
- If the oral cavity has blood, check for basal skull fracture, nasal or oral trauma, tongue laceration or/and injury or avulsion of teeth (Figure 9).
- Irrigate with saline. Administer antibiotics.
- Preserve loose tooth for re-implantation.
- Call for urgent ophthalmologic and plastic surgeon, if the face, eye or mouth are injured.

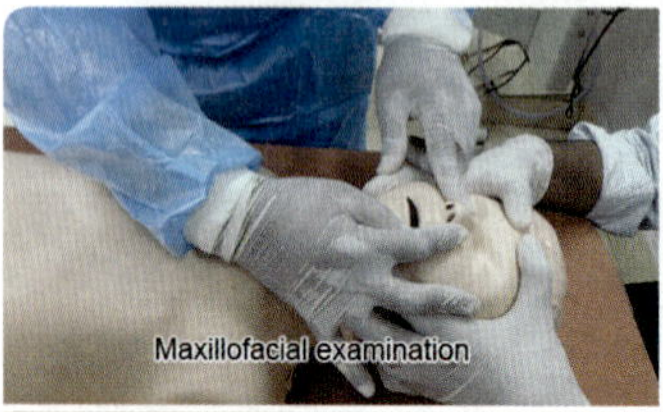

Figure 8: Examination of face and mouth.

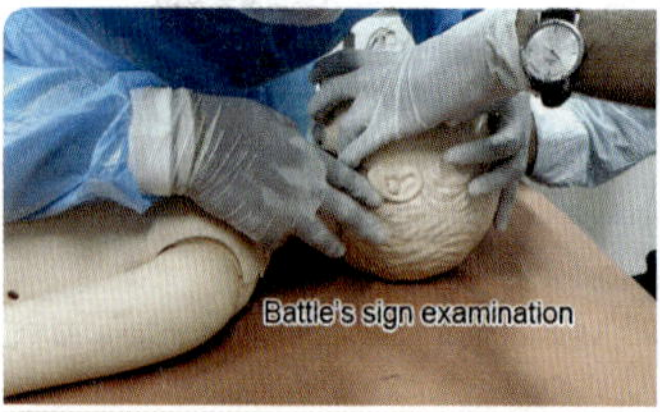

Figure 9: Examination of ears and mastoid for injury and bleed.
Note: Jaw thrust is being maintained.

Neck (Figure 10)

- Since the short necks of infants are difficult to assess, we can safely presume that an active child moving all four limbs is unlikely to have cervical cord injury.
- Maintain C-spine precaution in the unresponsive child or infant.

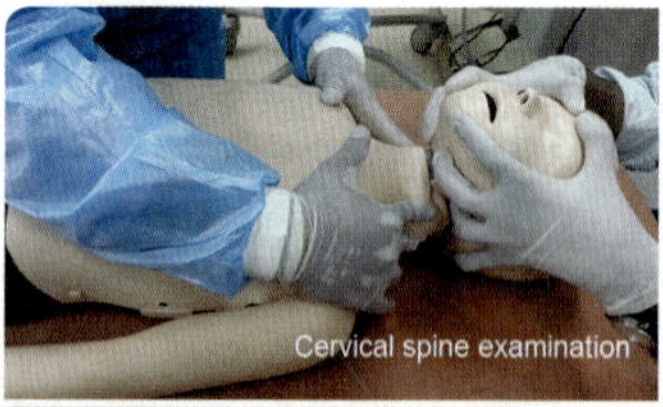

Figure 10: Examination of the neck.

Chest (Figures 11 to 14)

- Fracture of ribs and, therefore, flail chest is not common in young children.
- Initial chest X-ray may not show evidence of lung contusion.

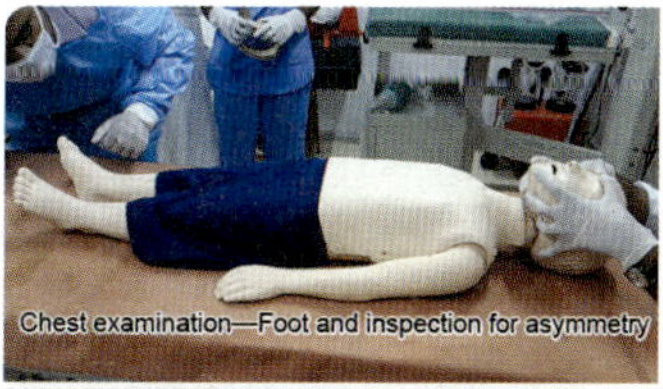

Figure 11: Examination of the chest for symmetry from the foot end of the victim.

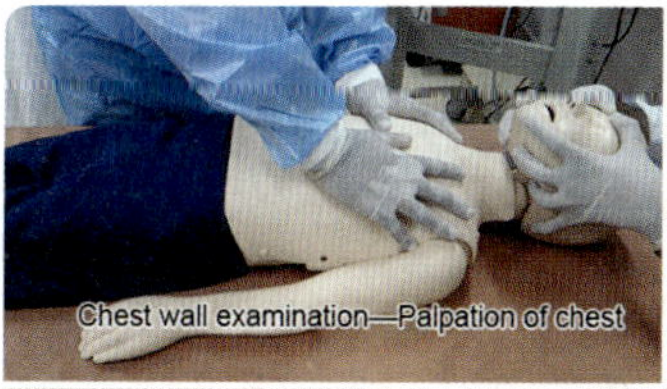

Figure 12: Palpation of the ribs and chest for soft tissue swelling and fracture of the ribs.

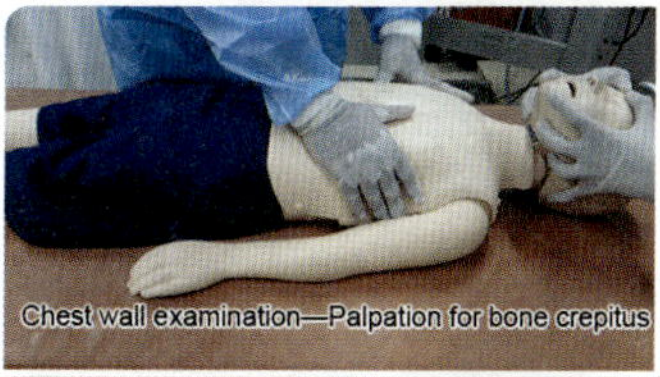

Figure 13: Palpation of ribs for bony crepitus.

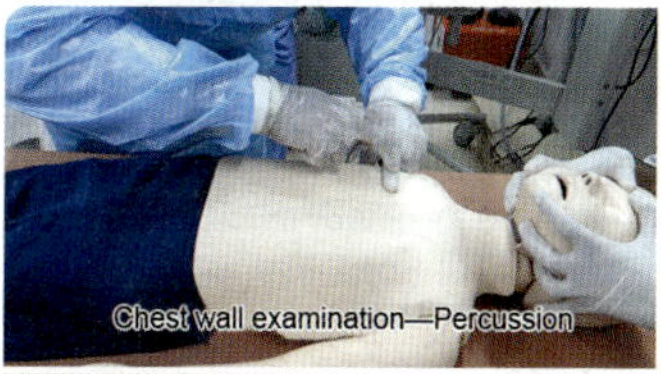

Figure 14: Percussion of chest for dullness or resonance. Resonance is suggestive of pneumothorax. Dullness is indicative of hemothorax.

Abdomen (Figure 15)

- Spleen and liver—refer to section on Abdominal and Pelvic trauma.

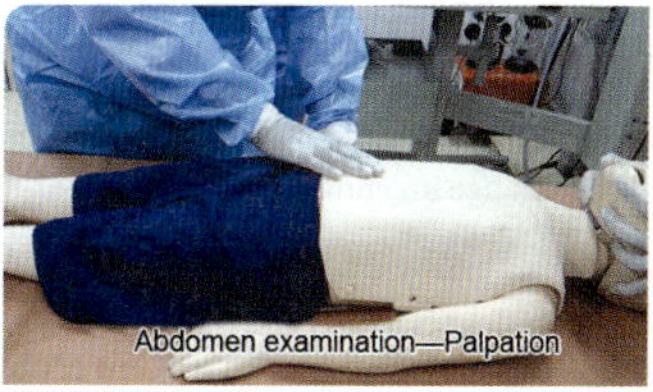

Figure 15: Examination of abdomen.

Perineum/Rectum/Vagina (Figure 16)

- Inspection of the perineum and the orifices give information on pelvic trauma

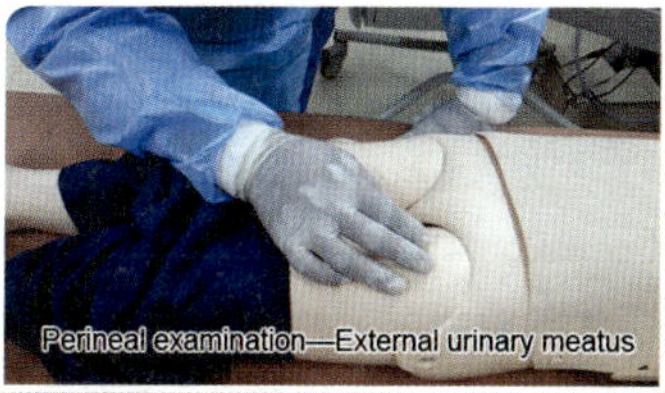

Figure 16: Examination of perineum.

(more common in children than in adults).
- Blood in the vagina or rectum warrants examination under anesthesia.

Unless blood is seen in the orifices, speculum examination need not be routinely performed in the pre-pubertal girl.

Neurological Evaluation

- Altered mental status due to hypoxia and shock may prevent accurate evaluation of the neurological status.
- Emesis may suggest raised intracranial pressure.
- Loss of tone, flaccidity and loss of sensation warrant neurosurgical consultation.
- However, lower spinal injuries are uncommon in children.

Interventions During Secondary Survey

- Antibiotics are administered for fractures, craniofacial injuries and abdominal trauma.
- Tetanus prophylaxis.
- Analgesia:
  - Morphine (0.1 mg/kg/dose).
  - Fentanyl (1 μg/kg/dose).
  - Paracetamol (15 mg/kg/dose PO/PR/NG).

Steroids not warranted for suspected spinal cord injury.

Circulation

- Apply direct pressure over open wounds.
- Simultaneously, realign the injured limb or limbs in the near anatomic position.
- Splint injured limbs.

Disability

- Assess gross motor function and circulation of each limb during the primary survey (Figures 17 and 18).

Move the deformed limb as little as possible

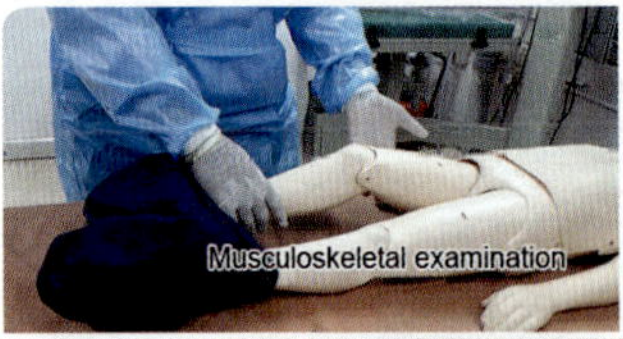

Figure 17: Examination of musculoskeletal system.

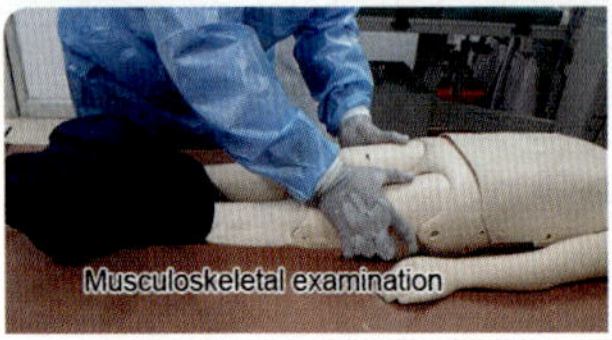

Figure 18: Examination of the muscles and the long bones for fracture or hematoma.

- Early splinting is the best analgesic.
- Avoid eliciting fracture crepitus.
- Remove the spinal board after spinal injuries have been ruled out by thorough neurological, radiological and magnetic resonance imaging (MRI) assessment.

Look, Feel, Move

Use your fingers to feel and move:
- From sternum and scapula to finger tips.
- From anterior superior iliac spine to toes.

- Examine pelvis for shape, tenderness, horizontal and vertical stability.
- Horizontal stability assessed by medial followed by lateral pressure on both anterior superior iliac spines (Figure 19).
- Vertical stability assessed by traction on one leg at a time, while stabilizing the pelvis.

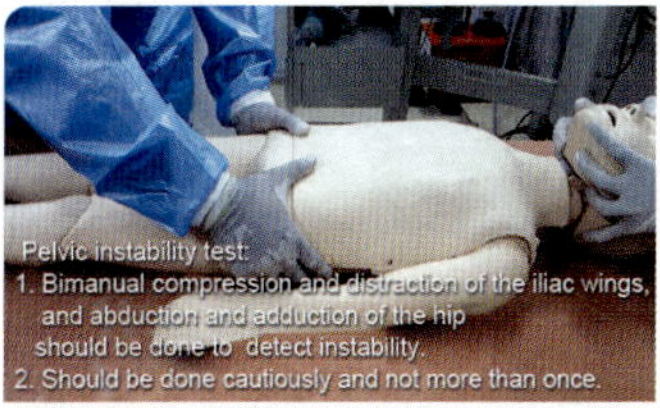

Figure 19: Pelvic stability test.

Pelvic fractures can cause exsanguinating bleed.

- Bind the pelvis circumferentially with a sheet to decrease its internal volume.
- Refer early for orthopedic intervention.
- Pelvic injury often associated with abdominal trauma. Laparotomy may be needed and may be performed along with pelvic stabilization

Examine an unstable pelvis only once. Repeated assessments could disrupt a clot and lead to blood loss. Bind the pelvis with a cloth/sheet to reduce volume and motion.

Spinal Injury

Palpate cervical spine for tenderness

- A fully conscious child, who is cooperative, can be requested to turn his head in all directions after removing the collar.
- Log roll the child and inspect and palpate the thoracic and lumbar spine up to the sacrum. Signs of injury include: (Figure 20)
  - Tenderness
  - Bruising
  - Swelling
  - Deformity (Figure 21).

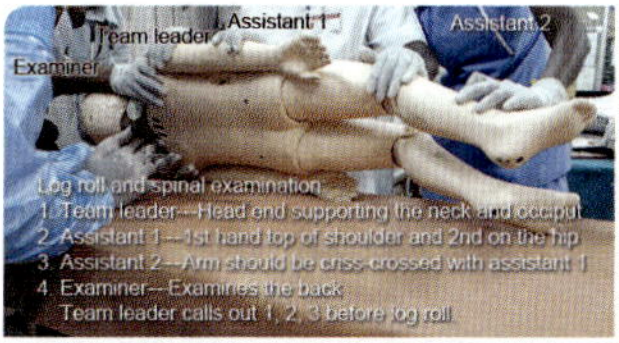

Figure 20: Technique of log rolling. The process, needs minimum 4 trained hands.

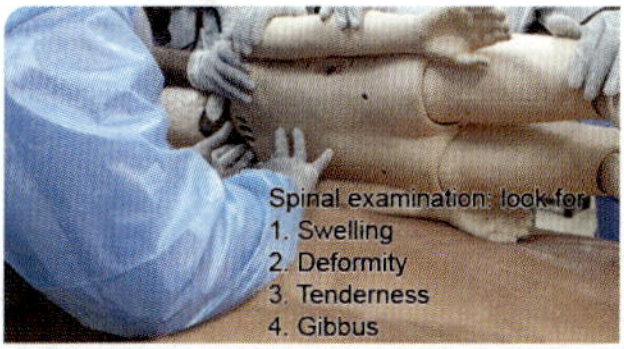

Figure 21: Application of spinal board during log roll. Spinal examination during log roll: Look for swelling, deformity, tenderness and gibbus. Note, the on-going support for the neck during log roll and spinal examination.

APPLICATION OF SPINAL BOARD (FIGURES 22 TO 26)

> *Boggy swelling over the lumbar spinous process or seat belt bruise denotes seat belt injury to spine.*

However, multiple injuries may be difficult to diagnose when the child is not alert or in pain. On the contrary, after a careful initial examination, a repeat physical examination at 24 hours or when the child becomes alert minimizes chances of missing injuries. Commonly missed injuries in motor vehicle accidents are fractures of metatarsal, tarsal, metacarpal and carpal bones.

> *Examine and document presence or absence of radial, ulnar, dorsalis pedis and posterior tibial pulses in all four limbs, whether the limb appears injured or not. Document color, temperature and motor function of all four limbs.*

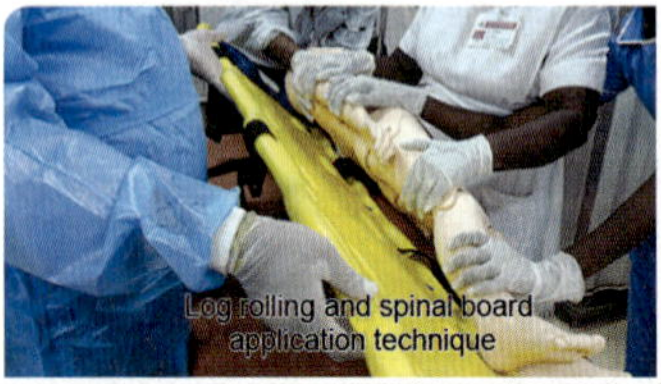

Figure 22: Method of application of spinal board during log roll without aggravating spinal injury.

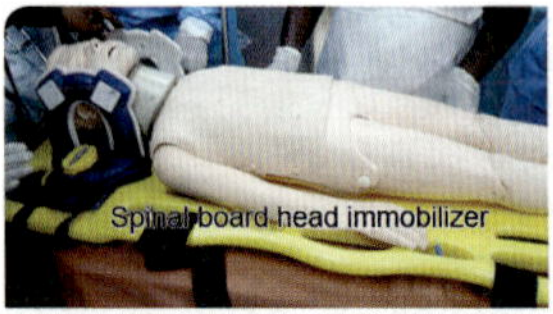

Figure 23: Application of head immobilizer along with the spinal board.

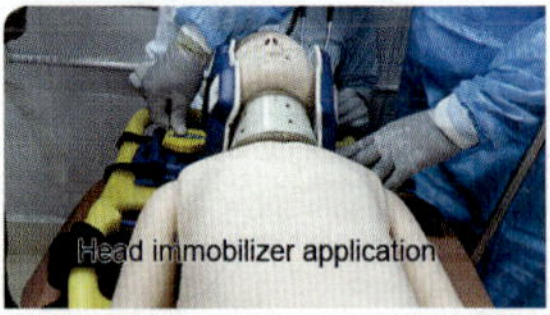

Figure 24: Method of application of spinal immobilizer, after application of cervical collar.

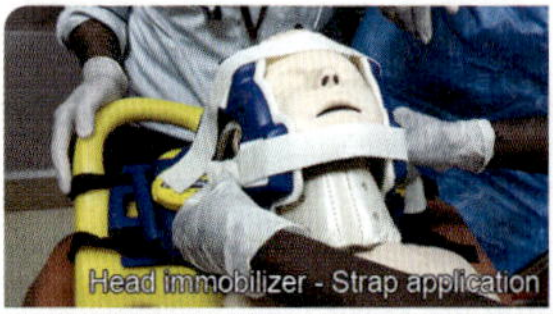

Figure 25: Fixing the head to the head immobilizer with straps provided for the purpose.

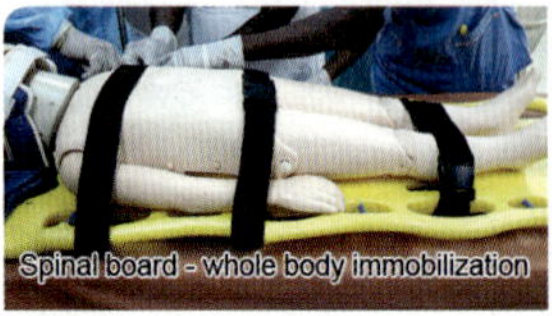

Figure 26: Whole body immobilization using straps. The straps are placed over the chest, anterior iliac spine and over the knees.

Neurological Examination (Table 1)

Evaluation of the power of each muscle according to the Medical Research Council (MRC) classification establishes whether the nerve is intact along its course. Younger children may be examined by observation using toys.

0 = No movement
1 = Flicker
2 = Moves without gravity (gravity eliminated)
3 = Moves with gravity (against gravity)
4 = Weaker than full strength
5 = Full strength

Table 1: Neurological examination

Nerve	Sensory	Motor
Radial nerve	First dorsal web space	Thumb extension, extension across MCP joints
Median nerve	Ulnar border of the index finger	Thumb opposition
Ulnar nerve	Tip of small finger	Abduction of index finger
Anterior interosseous nerve	N/A	Flexion of DIP joint of index finger and thumb
Peroneal nerve	Deep branch—first dorsal web space	Great toe dorsiflexion
Tibial nerve	Sole of foot at metatarsal heads	Ankle and toe plantar flexion

Open Wounds with or without Open Fractures

- Surface irrigation with saline.
- Apply sterile dressing.
- Administer antibiotics (Table 2).
- Tetanus prophylaxis.

Tetanus toxoid is administered if the child has not to be immunized as per the national immunization schedule or if he is older than 5 years (booster dose would have been given). Tetanus immunoglobulin 250–500 IU is administered if the victim has not been immunized and the wound is contaminated.

Suspect abdominal injury if secondary survey reveals the following:

- Abdominal distension.
- Abdominal tenderness.
- Abrasions.
- Ecchymosis.

Table 2: The Gustilo classification of open fractures to decide on antibiotic prophylaxis

Gustilo grade	Soft tissue injury	Antibiotic prophylaxis
I	Small laceration < 1 cm	Cefazolin 40 mg/kg
II	Laceration 1–10 cm, graft or flaps needed to cover	If penicillin/cef allergy: clindamycin 10 mg/kg
III a	Large laceration > 10 cm, extensive degloving injury, but bone can be covered	Cefazolin 40 mg/kg IV with gentamicin 2.5 mg/ kg IV with metronidazole 10 mg/kg if grossly contaminated (fecal, soil) or devitalized tissue
III b	Large laceration, bone cannot be covered, often extensive contamination	10 mg/kg clindamycin if pen/cef allergy
III c	Open fracture with arterial injury in same limb	10 mg/kg clindamycin if pen/cef allergy

Suspect serious abdominal trauma if infants are having predominantly chest breathing or the older child is lying still and whimpering or has referred pain to the shoulder. Trauma to the lower six ribs or abdominal distension in a hemodynamically unstable child is also associated with serious intra-abdominal injury.

Linear ecchymosis 'seat belt injury' is often associated with intra-abdominal injury.

Whilst abdominal X-ray is not useful in evaluation of intra-abdominal injury, radiographic evidence of gas in soft tissue (taken after stabilization) may provide some clues suggestive of bowel injury.

Splenic Injury

- Left shoulder pain (Kehr's sign).
- Abrasions and tenderness in left upper quadrant.
- Abdominal distension.
- Associated with shock.

Hepatic Injury

- Abdominal distension.
- Right shoulder pain.
- Abrasions and tenderness in right side of abdomen.
- Hypotensive shock.
- Injuries to the ribs are common.

Urological Injury

- Blood at penile meatus.
- Perineal bruising or swelling.
- High riding prostate.

If any of these signs are present, DO NOT insert a Foley's catheter. Diagnosis is confirmed by performing a retrograde urethrogram.

Transfer for imaging ONLY after stabilization.

Abdominal X-ray is not useful in evaluation of intra-abdominal injury,

Plain X-rays ordered for initial trauma survey are:

- Lateral C-spine.
- Chest.
- Pelvis.
- Two views at 90° for injured limb segments and spine.
- Include the joint above and below the injured segment.

Computed Tomography (CT) Scan

- Useful if complex flat bone trauma, such as pelvis, spinal injuries are suspected.

Magnetic Resonance Imaging (MRI)

- Does not play a major role in management of orthopedic injuries.
- Indicated if clinical signs of spinal cord injury are noted.

Major exsanguinating trauma:

Plan to urgently shift to the operation theater for damage control surgery.

KEY POINTS

1. Rushing to evaluate obvious injuries, with failure to stabilize the ABCs is a common error in the management of trauma.
2. Stabilization and immobilization of the spine is a priority in trauma victims
3. Rule out hemo/pneumothorax and control bleeding in addition to stabilization of the ABCs.
4. Ensure comfort for children who do not have life-threatening injuries.
5. MRI not a useful modality in orthopedic trauma.
6. FAST mandatory in ruling out intra-abdominal bleed.
7. Manually immobilize C-spine until the cervical collar and spinal board has been applied.
8. Shift to OT when shock is refractory to fluid therapy.
9. Do not transfer trauma victim for imaging without stabilization.
10. Infusing whole blood early in the management of exsanguinating bleed due to trauma.

BURNS

BURNS CLASSIFICATION

Burns classification is based on depth, extent and involvement of hands or face or perineum.

1. First degree/superficial
   - Red, dry painful.
   - Will heal after a few days with no scar.
2. Second degree/partial thickness
   - Wet, red, very painful.
   - Superficial or deep partial thickness.
   - Will heal by scar (may require skin graft).
   - Needs wound care and possible debridement, but will heal after weeks.
3. Third degree/full thickness
   - Leathery, dry, loss of sensation, waxy.
   - Will heal with excision and grafting.
4. Fourth degree
   - Involves subcutaneous tissue, tendon and bone.

Pre-hospital Care

Do not remove burned clothing.

- Make sure the victim is no longer in contact with hot or burning material or exposed to smoke or heat.
- Cool the area within 30 minutes of the burn with cool water. This intervention reduces the depth of burnt area and pain.

Do not put ICE on the Burn

1. Do not immerse large severe burns in ice cold water. Doing so could cause a drop in body temperature (hypothermia) and deterioration of blood pressure and circulation (shock).
2. Cover the area of the burn. Use a cool, moist, sterile bandage; clean, moist cloth; or moist cloth towels.
3. Elevate the burned body part or parts above heart level, when possible.

Airway and Breathing

- Provide oxygen to spontaneously breathing victim
- If not breathing, initiate bag valve mask ventilation and plan early intubation.

Consider early intubation if the following signs are noted:

- Singed nasal hairs and eyebrows.
- Carbonaceous deposits in oropharynx and face.
- Oropharyngeal edema.
- Hoarseness, persistent coughing, stridor.
- Face, neck, upper torso burns.
- Aspiration of hot liquids can also cause airway compromise.
- Anticipate a difficult airway and call for ENT or anesthesiologist help and use a smaller size ET tube.

Circulation

- Two large peripheral intravenous lines should be obtained.

- Correct shock with normal saline (NS) boluses (Figure 27).
- If the child has suffered inhalation injuries along with skin burns, 40–50% more fluid may be warranted.

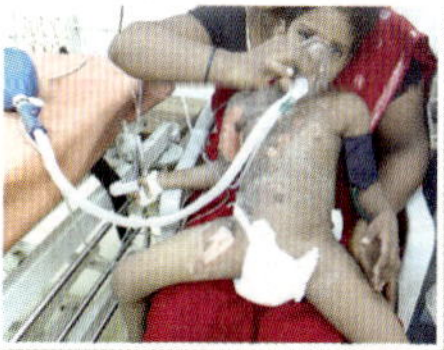

Figure 27: O_2, NS bolus, Dopamine and Norepinephrine infusions were needed for resolution of cardiogenic shock following burns.

Total Burn Surface Area (Table 3)

- Calculate using rule of nine (Refer to Figure 28)
- Exclude first-degree burns when calculating total burn surface area.

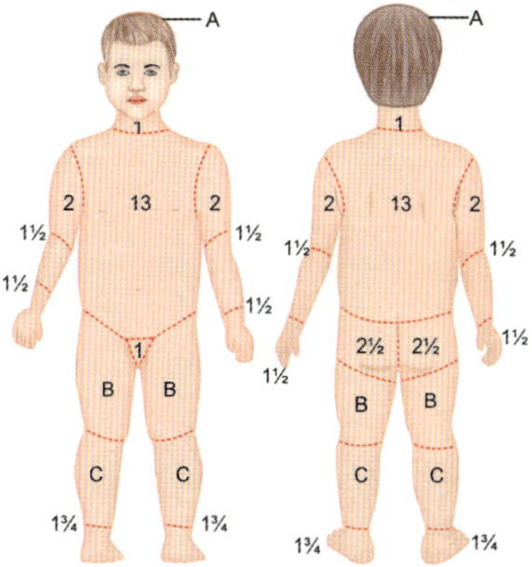

A = half of head

B = half of one thigh

C = half of one lower leg

Age	0	1	5	10	15
A	9½	8½	6½	5½	4½
B	2¾	4	4½	4½	4¾
C	2½	2¾	3	3¾	3½

Figure 28: Surface area for infants

Table 3: Burns estimate—age versus area

	Birth–1 year	1–4 years	5–9 years	10–14 years	15 years	2°	3°	Total
Head	19	17	13	11	9			
Neck	2	2	2	2	2			
Anterior trunk	13	13	13	13	13			
Posterior trunk	13	13	13	13	13			
Right buttock	2 ½	2½	2½	2½	2½			
Left buttock	2½	2½	2½	2½	2½			
Genitalia	1	1	1	1	1			
Right upper arm	4	4	4	4	4			
Left upper arm	4	4	4	4	4			
Right lower arm	3	3	3	3	3			
Left lower arm	3	3	3	3	3			
Right hand	2½	2½	2½	2½	2½			
Left hand	2½	2½	2½	2½	2½			
Right thigh	5½	6½	8	8½	9			
Left thigh	5½	6½	8	8½	9			
Right leg	5	5	5½	6	6½			
Left leg	5	5	5½	6	6½			
Right foot	3½	3½	3½	3½	3½			
Left foot	3½	3½	3½	3½	3½			

Parkland Resuscitation Formula

4 mL/kg of fluids/% total burn surface area.

- Time zero for fluid resuscitation = Time of burn injury.
- Total fluids to be given for first 24 hours = Normal maintenance for age + 4 mL/kg/% total body surface area.
- Give half of calculated fluids over first 8 hours from time of injury.
- Give remaining half of calculated volume over the following 16 hours.
- Do not forget on-going losses, such as vomiting.
- Adjust fluids to maintain output of 1–2 mL/kg/hour.
- Loss of albumin in open wounds could result in hypoalbuminemia. However, during resuscitation, albumin is not advised.
- Tetanus prophylaxis
- Avoid prophylactic antibiotics.
- Provide pain relief.
- Intravenous antibiotics are recommended only in large and severe burns.

CARE OF BURNED OR SCALDED AREA

Scalds

Scald burns do not require surgery. Wound cleansing and dressing changes are sufficient (Figures 29 A to D).

Facial Burns

- Rule out corneal injury.
- Lubricate if eye lids are swollen

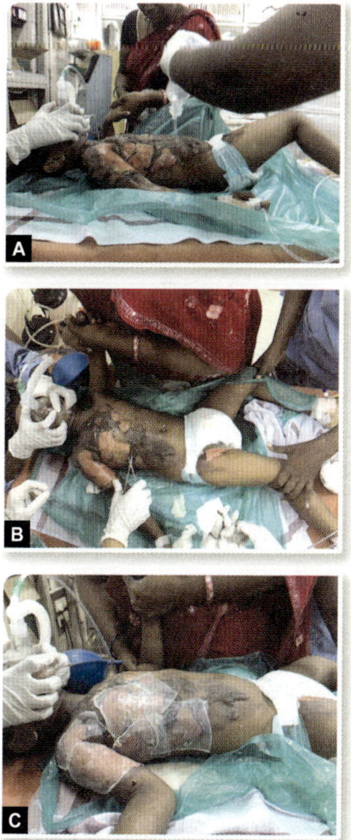

Figures 29A to C: Care of the burns area in the emergency department: (A) Provide oxygen and correct shock, (B) Debride the necrotic and burned tissue. (Remember to provide pain relief by administering rectal paracetamol and fentanyl infusion throughout the procedure), (C) Application of collagen after debridement.

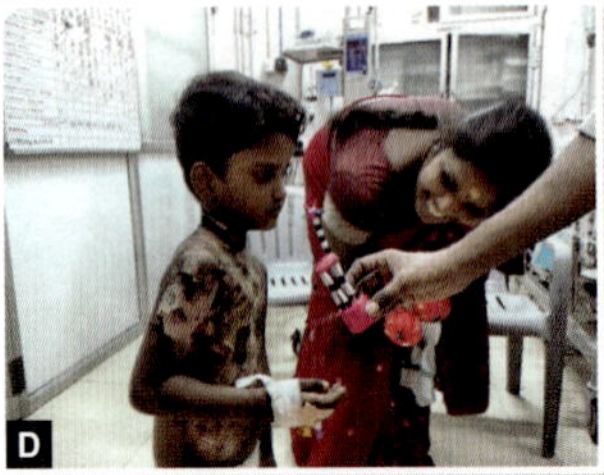

Figure 29D: Complete recovery following correc-tion of shock and burns management in the PED.

- Secure ET tube with wire if extensive facial involvement

Scalp Burns

- Shave hair to assess extent of burns
- Keep wound clean

Hand Burns

- Meticulous wound cleaning and dressing
- Plastic surgery follow up is essential to avoid contractures

Commissure Burns (Burns Around Mouth)

Warn parents the potential for late bleeding. (Labial artery can get exposed when eschar separates after 5 to 10 days).

Burn Specific Secondary Survey

- Rule out intra-cranial trauma
- Corneal fluorescein exam for corneal injury
- Assess for burns and exposed cartilage
- Circumferential burns around chest may warrant escharotomy
- Abdominal compartment syndrome could occur
- Check foreskin for genitourinary injury
- Pain during passive/voluntary movements (consider escharotomy if circumferential burns)

Investigations

- CBC, electrolytes and renal function should be evaluated
- Chest X-ray

KEY POINTS

1. Wash burned areas with tap water in the pre-hospital setting.
2. Anticipating need for early intubation, if airway is involved.
3. Estimation of burned surface and calculating the appropriate fluids.
4. Estimate the size of the burned surface for calculating fluid requirements.

11

CHAPTER

Approach to Fever in Children

Chapter Outline

- Acute Gastroenteritis
- Lower Respiratory Tract Infections (LRTIs)
- Typhoid Fever
- Management of Diphtheria

FEVER IS THE MOST COMMON CAUSE FOR HOSPITAL VISITS

Causes: Common

1. Viral fever
2. URI
3. Typhoid
4. Para-typhoid
5. Malaria
6. Pneumonia
7. UTI
8. Dengue illness
9. Scrub typhus
10. Enteritis
11. TB

Uncommon Causes

1. Sinusitis
2. Otitis media
3. Abscess
4. Extended viral fever
5. Infectious mononucleosis
6. Osteomyelitis
7. Endocarditis
8. Leptospirosis
9. Collagen vascular diseases and malignancy

STEP 1: IS IT VIRAL OR BACTERIAL OR PROTOZOAL (MALARIA)?

Recognize Viral Infection: Use of Antibiotics can cause more Harm than Good!

- Viral fever, typically, starts as high-grade fever that resolves by day 3 or 4
- Child does not appear "sick"
- The inter-febrile period is normal
- Focus of infection: Not often clear. May have evidence of upper respiratory infection, pharyngeal congestion or rashes
- More than one contact

Treatment: Anti-pyretics

- Avoid antibiotics

Bacterial Infection

- Fever is initially moderate, peaking by day 3 or 4
- Child appears sick.
- The inter-febrile period is usually not normal
- Focus: Visual evidence of infection is usually apparent (otitis, impetigo, UTI, etc.)
- No sick contacts

STEP 2: IS THIS FEBRILE EPISODE HARMLESS OR DANGEROUS (SEPSIS)?

Ask mom the following questions:

1. Does her child have history of incessant cry, lethargy, is more sleepy, or as usual or not?
2. Breathless? (not episodic or since birth)

STEP 3: PLAN OF ACTION

No → Alert (not toxic); Yes → Fall in mental status

	Alert (not toxic)	Fall in mental status
1.	Social smile	No smile, vacant look, not interested in surroundings (responsive to voice)
2.	Consolable	Inconsolable cry (responsive to voice)
3.	Playful, making eye contact	Not smiling at mom (responsive to pain)
4.	Active	Floppy or lethargic (responsive to pain)
5.	Quiet	Moaning or grunting (responsive to pain)

↓ Urgent resuscitation is needed.

↓ Anticipate septic cardiogenic shock. Perform rapid cardiopulmonary cerebral assessment.

	0–1 Month	1–3 Months	3–36 Months
Abnormal appearance, increased respiratory rates, flushed color.	Cardiopulmonary cerebral assessment Management of septic cardiogenic shock if identified Sepsis screen Empirical antibiotics		
Alert playful, normal respiratory rates, pink	Hospitalization Sepsis screen Empirical antibiotics	Treatment guided by CBC, CRP, smear for malaria, urine screen	CBC, CRP only if fever > 103°F

ANTIPYRETICS AND ANALGESICS

Paracetamol

Oral	10–15 mg/kg/dose 4–6 hourly
Rectal	10–20 mg/kg/dose 4–6 hourly
IV	10–15 mg/kg/dose 6–8 hourly
Overdose (poisonous)	**> 150 mg/kg => Fatal hepatic necrosis**
Antidote	N-Acetylcysteine

Ibuprofen

Oral	5–10 mg/kg/dose 6–8 hourly Max 40 mg/kg/day
Caution	**Can precipitate GI bleed especially in Dengue fever, Asthma in at-risk children, not to be used in infants < 6 months.**
Ideally indicated in the following conditions	Juvenile rheumatoid arthritis PDA closure in preemies

Mefenamic Acid

Fever	3 mg/kg/dose
Arthritis	25–30 mg/kg/day 6–8 hourly

Caution—Colitis, Thrombocytopenia

Peptic ulcers, renal and liver impairment
Not advisable since it carries increased risk of the following side effects:

Diclofenac Sodium—NSAIDs are not recommended for fever in children.

Rational choice of antibiotics is based on the causative organisms.

Antibiotics, if wrongly used, cause more harm than good!

Site of infection	Likely organism	Choice of antibiotic	
		First line drugs	Second line drugs
Acute pharyngitis	Group A Beta Hemolytic Streptococcus	✓ 1st generation – Cephalosporin ✓ Penicillin V	✓ Macrolides
Acute otitis media, Acute sinusitis	S. pneumoniae H. influenzae B M. cattarhalis	✓ Amoxycillin	✓ Co-amoxyclav ✓ 2nd generation Cephalosporin ✓ Macrolides
Acute epiglottitis	H Influenzae	✓ Ceftriaxone	✓ Cefotaxime ✓ Ampicillin + sulbactam
Lower respiratory infections			
< 3 months	Gram (–)ve Infection, H. influenzae B Staphylococcus	✓ Cefotaxime or Ceftriaxone +/– Aminoglycoside ✓ Cloxacillin or ✓ Vancomycin or ✓ Linezolid (if Staphylococcus)	
3 months – 5 years	H. influenzae B S. pneumoniae Staphylococcus	✓ Amoxycillin ✓ Co-amoxyclav or ✓ 2nd generation Cephalosporins (Cefuroxime)	✓ Co-amoxyclav ✓ Ceftriaxone or ✓ Cefotaxime
> 5 Years	S. pneumoniae Mycoplasma pneumoniae	✓ Penicillin ✓ Amoxycillin/ ✓ Co-amoxyclav ✓ Macrolides	✓ Cefuroxime ✓ Ceftriaxone or ✓ Cefotaxime AND Macrolides (Clarithromycin or Azithromycin)
Typhoid fever	Salmonella typhi S. paratyphi A	✓ 3rd generation oral Cephalosporin ✓ Azithromycin ✓ Fluoroquinolone	✓ 3rd generation oral/ inj. Cephalosporin ✓ Fluoroquinolone ✓ Chloramphenicol
Urinary tract infections	E. coli Proteus Klebsiella Pseudomonas Enterococci	✓ Fluoroquinolone ✓ Co-amoxyclav	✓ Aminoglycoside ✓ Fluoroquinolone ✓ Nitrofurantoin ✓ 3rd generation Cephalosporin
Skin and soft tissue infections	Staphylococcus Streptococcus	✓ Erythromycin ✓ Penicillin ✓ Amoxyclav	✓ Macrolides ✓ Cephalexin ✓ Cefadroxyl

KEY POINTS

1. Fever is not an indication for antibiotics.
2. Viral etiologies are the commonest cause of fever in children.
3. Antibiotics are indicated based on focus of infection.
4. Anticipate severe sepsis for every child with fever by asking triage questions and performing the rapid cardiopulmonary cerebral assessment.

ACUTE GASTROENTERITIS

Up to 30–50% of diarrhea are caused by Rota virus or enterotoxigenic E. coli (ETEC). Hence, antibiotics are not indicated in acute diarrhea.

Management: Low osmolarity ORS (245 mmol/L).

- 10 mL/kg for every episode of loose stool and vomiting.
- If child vomits or not taking enough: Give small sips of ORS.

Other Fluids used for Oral Rehydration

1. Food-based solutions:
   Rice water with salt, lassi with salt
2. Home-available solutions:
   Plain water, lemon water, coconut water, soups, thin rice, kanji, dal water.

What is NOT Oral Rehydrating Fluid?

1. Glucose water without salt
2. Fluids without salt or sugar
3. Fluids in small quantity

Zinc: Decreases the frequency as well as recurrence of diarrhea

Zinc Sulphate, Zinc Acetate (or) Zinc Gluconate

- $>$ 6 months old—20 mg/day OD (or) BD
- $<$ 6 months—10 mg/day (10 to 14 days)

Avoid Iron-Containing Formula

Antibiotics are indicated if:

1. Cholera
2. Bloody diarrhea (shigellosis)
3. Serious associated non-GIT infections (pneumonia, sepsis, meningitis, UTI)
4. Infants < 3 months
5. SAM

ANTI-MICROBIALS

1.	Ciprofloxacin (Ofloxacin and Norfloxacin can be used)	15 mg/kg twice a day – 3 days
2.	Cefixime	8 mg/kg/day – 5 days
3.	Ceftriaxone	50–100 mg/kg OD – 2 days
4.	Azithromycin	6–20 mg/kg OD – 1–5 days

Drugs not effective in diarrhea:

1. Aminoglycosides, Nitrofurans, Nalidixic acid, Metronidazole (***Metronidazole can cause nausea and vomiting and worsen the dehydration***).

Amoebiasis is less common in children less than 5 years of age.

2. Anti-motility drugs: Loperamide.

KEY POINTS

1. ORS is the mainstay of therapy for acute diarrhea.
2. Zinc therapy is recommended along with ORS.
3. Antibiotics are not routinely indicated.

LOWER RESPIRATORY TRACT INFECTIONS (LRTIs)

Age	First line	Alternatives
3 months–5 years	Amoxicillin 30–50 mg/kg/day	Coamoxiclav–40 mg/kg/day Cefuroxime–20–30 mg/kg/day Chloramphenicol
> 5 years	Amoxicillin	Azithromycin (10 mg/kg/day) or Clarithromycin (15 mg/kg/day)/ Coamoxyclav/Cefuroxime

KEY POINTS

1. **Normal saline nasal drops** are much more helpful than anti-histaminics for nasal congestion and nasal discharge.
2. **Anti-histaminics** cause crust formation and block the airway
3. **Anti-histamines are indicated for symptoms of allergy:** Sneezing, itching.
4. **Third generation cephalosporin: Cefixime is not useful in the management of respiratory tract infections.**

TYPHOID FEVER

1.	Cefixime	20 mg/kg/day bd 14 days
2.	Azithromycin	20 mg/kg/day od 7 days
3.	Inj. Cefotaxime	150 mg/kg/day tds 14 days
4.	Inj. Ceftriaxone	50–75 mg/kg/day bd 14 days
5.	Ciprofloxacin or Ofloxacin (Drug-resistant typhoid)	10–15 mg/kg/day bd

MALARIA

	Drug sensitivity	Recommended treatment
1.	P. vivax and chloroquine sensitive P. falciparum	Chloroquine 10 mg base/kg stat followed by 5 mg/kg at 6, 24 and 48 hrs OR Chloroquine 10 mg base/kg stat followed by 10 mg/kg at 24 hrs and 5 mg/kg at 48 hrs (total dose 25 mg base/kg)
2.	P. vivax	T. primaquine 0.25 mg/kg OD for 14 days
3.	P. falciparum	T. primaquine 0.75 mg/kg single dose
4.	Chloroquine-resistant P. falciparum	T. artesunate 4 mg/kg OD for 3 days and Sulfadoxine 25 mg/kg and Pyrimethamine 1.5 mg/kg OD single dose on Day 1

URINARY TRACT INFECTION (UTI)

- Can present without obvious focus
- Vomiting may be sole symptom

Male child:

- Check out posterior urethral valve by looking for good stream of urine
- Look for phimosis.

A clean catch sample from first void specimen is sent for analysis. The sample is obtained midstream.

Laboratory Diagnosis of UTI

- Mild proteinuria
- Leukocyturia, > 5 leucocytes/high power field in a centrifuged specimen OR > 10 leucocytes/high power field in an uncentrifuged sample
- Bacteria on Gram stain
- Positive leucocyte esterase and nitrite tests by dipstick.

Culture positive UTI: Further work-up is mandatory. Imaging is needed to identify reflux (Early recognition of UTI is essential to prevent renal scaring).

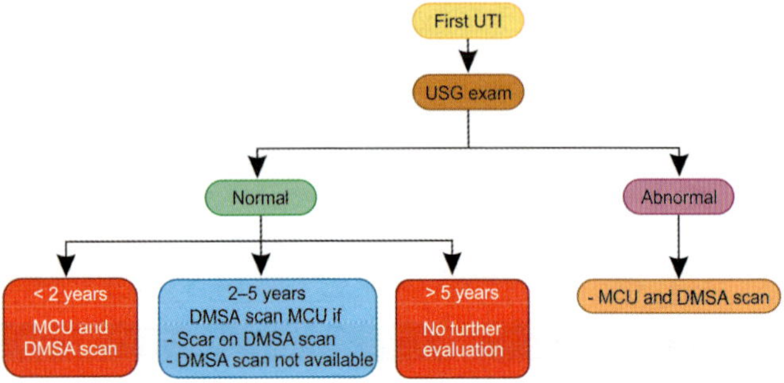

MCU: Micturation cysto-urethrogram, DMSA: Dimercaptosuccinic acid scan

SCRUB TYPHUS

Fever, eschar (diagnostic), hepatosplenomegaly, lymphadenopathy, thrombocytopenia.

1.	Doxycycline	5 mg/kg/day bd – 5–7 days (or) 3 days of afebrile period.
2.	Azithromycin	10 mg/kg/ OD – 5–7 days

SKIN AND SOFT TISSUE INFECTIONS

Staphylococcus and streptococci are the commonest causative organisms.
Local care: Cleansing, removal of crusts, wet dressings

Topical Treatment

1.	Mupirocin	2% 2 times/day for 7–10 days
2.	Fusidic acid	2% 2–5 times/day
3.	Systemic antibiotics (if widespread, peri-oral, deep involvement)	
Cephalexin/cefadroxil/cloxacillin/amoxiclav/erythromycin/ Azithromycin If MRSA: Clindamycin/cotrimoxazole, linezolid		5–7 days
	Don't use cefixime, (not effective against S. aureus)	

Scabies

1.	Permethrin	2.5% to 5% dermal cream Wash after 12 hrs. 2nd application after a week Avoid in infants <2 months
2.	Gamma benzene hexachloride	Avoid in children with history of seizures Contraindicated in children <5 years or weighing <15 kg
3.	Oral ivermectin	3–6 mg single dose

MANAGEMENT OF DIPHTHERIA

1. Specimen for culture should be obtained from nose, throat and muco-cutaneous lesions. A portion of membrane should be removed and submitted with underlying exudates.
2. Strict bed rest
3. Horse Diphtheritic Anti-serum
4. Antibiotics
   Inj. Crystalline penicillin 1–1.5 lakh units/kg/day in four divided doses for 14 days
   Or
   Oral Erythromycin 50 mg/kg/day in four divided doses for 14 days
5. Active immunization of the child
   DPT < 7 years
   Td > 7 years
6. Intubation and mechanical ventilation if there is upper airway obstruction, resection of pseudomembrane if needed

TETANUS/GAS GANGRENE

1. Meticulous supportive care:
   a. Quite dark secluded setting
   b. Minimal handling
   c. Tracheostomy kit to be ready
   d. Maintenance of fluid, electrolyte and calorie balance
   e. Constant and meticulous nursing attention to mouth, bladder, bowel and skin
2. Surgical Wound Excision
3. Tetanus Immuoglobulin (TIG) - 3,000 units IM or Tetanus Antitoxin – 50,000 – 1.0 lakh units IM or IV after test dose

Site	Dosage of Diphtheritic anti-serum
Pharyngeal or laryngeal disease of 48 hours or less duration	20,000 to 40,000 units
Nasopharyngeal < 48 hours	40,000 to 60,000 units
a. Extensive pharyngeal or b. Laryngeal diphtheria c. Brawny Swelling of the neck d. Disease longer than 48 hours	80,000 to 1,20,000 units
Cutaneous	20,000 to 40,000 units

Desensitization of Diphtheria Antitoxin—IV route

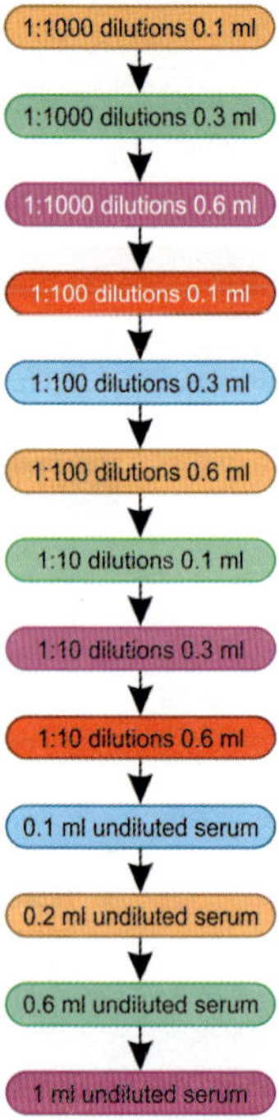

4. Antibiotics
   a. Penicillin G 1.0 lakh units/kg/day in 4–6 divided doses IV for 10–14 days
   b. IV Metronidazole 7.5 mg/kg/dose 8th hourly for 10–14 days
5. Anticonvulsants and Muscle relaxants

a. Diazepam drip: Inj. Diazepam 2.5 mg/kg dissolved in 100 mL of normal saline for every 12 hours (2 doses/day). The diazepam drip to be continued for 2 to 6 weeks after the spasms are controlled and then slowly tapered or Inj. Diazepam 0.2 mg/kg 3–6 hourly
b. Chlorpromazine can be added 2 mg/kg/24 hours in 4–6 divided doses orally if patient continues to have severe spasms
c. If the patient continues to have spasms the patient must be treated with mechanical ventilation.

BIBLIOGRAPHY

1. Tiwari TP, Clark T. Use of Diphtheria Antitoxin (DAT) for Suspected Diphtheria Cases, Centers for Disease Control and Prevention (CDC), 2014.

12
CHAPTER

Special Topics

Chapter Outline

- Prophylaxis
- How to Avoid Catastrophe During CT/MRI?

TETANUS PROPHYLAXIS IN WOUND MANAGEMENT

Vaccination history	Clean, minor wounds		All other wounds	
	TD	TIG	TD	TIG*
Unknown, < 3 doses, immunodeficient	Yes	No	Yes	Yes
> 3 doses	No**	No	No***	No

*TIG: Tetanus immunoglobulin (250–500 IU IM)
** Yes, if more than 10 years since last dose
*** Yes, if more than 5 years since last dose

RABIES EXPOSURE AND RECOMMENDED POST-EXPOSURE PROPHYLAXIS

Category	Type of contact	Type of exposure	Recommended Post-exposure prophylaxis (PEP)
I	Touching or feeding of animals. Licks on intact skin	None	None, if reliable case history is available
II	Nibbling of uncovered skin. Minor scratches or abrasions without bleeding	Minor	Wound management + Anti-rabies vaccine

Contd...

Contd...

Category	Type of contact	Type of exposure	Recommended Post-exposure prophylaxis (PEP)
III	Single or multiple transdermal bites or scratches, licks on broken skin Contamination of mucous membrane with saliva (i.e. licks)	Severe	Wound management + Rabies immunoglobulin + Anti-rabies vaccine

Measures to be Followed After a Dog Bite

Supportive Care

- Clean the wound thoroughly with soap and water. Subsequently, use 40 to 70% alcohol, or Betadine solution.
- Avoid suturing the wound.
- Depending on the immunization status of the child, order injection Tetanus Toxoid and Tetanus Immunoglobulin
- Antibiotics are recommended, only if the wounds are multiple or contaminated. The preferred antibiotic is Amoxycillin clavulinic acid.

Postexposure Prophylaxis

- Active immunoprophylaxis is provided using tissue culture vaccines given on days 0, 3, 7, 14 and 30 (day 90 dose optional). Day 0, is the date of commencement of the 1st dose.
- Bites from dogs, cats, cows, buffaloes, sheep, goats, pigs, donkeys, horses, camels, foxes, jackals, monkeys, mongoose, bear bites warrant PEP.
- Rabies have not been reported following rodent bites, such as rats and mice, etc. Hence, postexposure prophylaxis is not normally recommended for these bites.

HIV

PEP Recommendations

Occupational Exposure

Exposure codes	HIV source code	PEP recommendations	Duration
1	1	**Not warranted**	28 days
1	2	**Recommended**	
2	1		
2	2		
3	1 or 2		
2/3	Unknown	Consider PEP, if HIV prevalence is high in the given population and risk categorization	

HIV EXPOSURE CODE

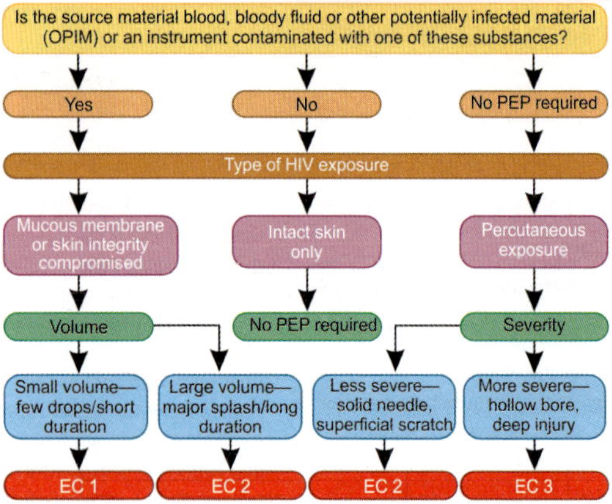

HIV SOURCE CODE

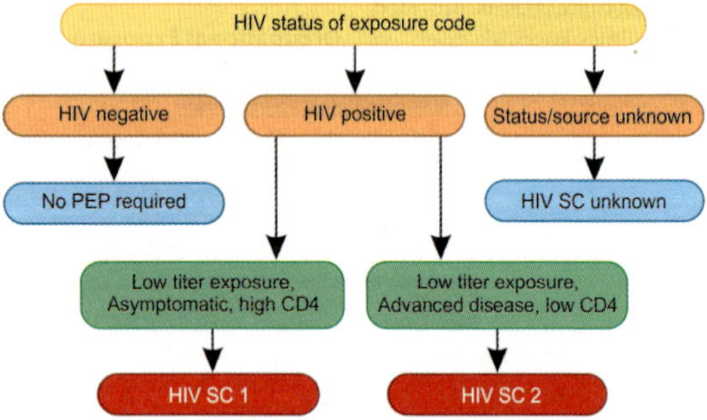

PEP Regimen

- Recommended regimen is Tenofovir 300 mg + Lamivudine 300 mg + Efavirenz 600 mg once daily for 28 days.
- Currently, postexposure prophylaxis regimen is available round the clock in all major hospitals.
- The first dose of PEP is administered as soon as possible, preferably within 2 hours of exposure. The subsequent dose is taken at bed time (2–3 hours after dinner). Fatty food is not advised while taking these drugs at bedtime.

HIV STATUS OF SOURCE OF EXPOSURE

Source of HIV	Definition of risk in source
HIV Negative	Source is not HIV-infected; but consider HBV and HCV
Low Risk	HIV positive and clinically asymptomatic
High Risk	HIV positive and clinically symptomatic
Unknown	Status of the patient unknown Neither patient nor his/her blood available for testing The risk assessment will be based only upon the exposure (HIV prevalence in the geographical area should be considered)

HOW TO AVOID CATASTROPHE DURING CT/MRI?

1. Children may need sedation during imaging. They may also need IV contrast for the same purpose. Unfortunately, sedation or anaphylaxis can precipitate cardiac arrest. This section deals with how we can prevent these catastrophes!
2. Ask triage questions to the mother
3. Perform and document the rapid cardiopulmonary cerebral assessment. Don't forget to document the time and date of your assessment!
4. Plan to shift only if the triage questions are negative and the physiological status is normal

If anaphylaxis occurs during IV contrast administration:

- *Administer epinephrine deep IM (anterolateral aspect of thigh)*
- *Dose of epinephrine:*
  - *12 yrs: 500 µg IM (0.5 mL), i.e. same as adult dose.*
  - *If child is small or prepubertal: 300 µg (0.3 mL).*
  - *6–12 yrs: 300 µg IM (0.3 mL).*
  - *6 months–6 yrs: 150 µg IM (0.15 mL).*
  - *< 6 months: 150 µg IM (0.15 mL).*

5. Carry the largest bag valve mask with age-appropriate mask. Reservoir is a must. The reservoir ensures that the bag valve mask device delivers 100% oxygen. Do not carry the bag valve mask device in your bag. It should be immediately available if the need arises (Figure 1).
6. Carry pre-filled epinehrine (1 mL of 1: 1000 is diluted in 9 mL NS) the bag valve mask device in your bag. It should be immedia-tely available if the need arises (Figure 1).
7. Ensure that the baby has a venflon through which emergency drugs may be administered.
8. Carry a prefilled 10 ml syringe with dilute Adrenaline (1:10000 dilution) pre-filled syringe. If contrast infusion causes anaphylactic shock, rapid administration of 0.1 ml/kg IV or deep IM (if IV access is unavailable) is mandatory.
9. Learn to recognize respiratory arrest and initiate bag valve mask ventilation.
10. Learn to administer age-appropriate chest compression.

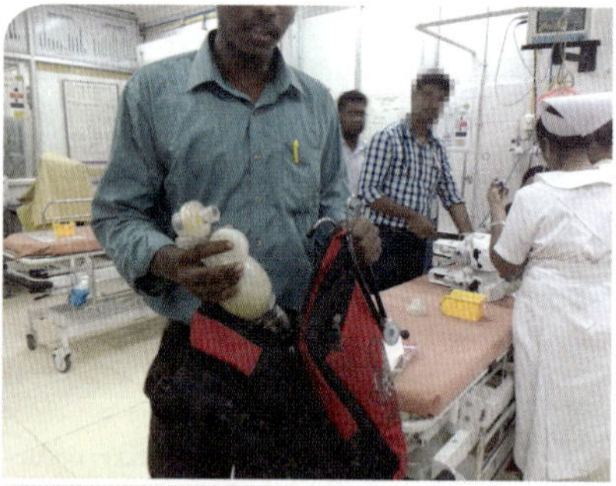

Figure 1: Note the intern is carrying a tiny bag valve mask device inside a bag. This can prevent rapid response to initiating breath for apnea due to midazolam.

KEY POINTS

1. Midazolam-induced respiratory arrest can lead to hypoxic ischemic encephalopathy or cardiac arrest.
2. Contrast-induced anaphylaxis can also result in cardiac arrest.
3. Cardiac arrest due to both disasters is potentially preventable.

13

CHAPTER

Clinical Skills

Chapter Outline

- Handwashing
- How to do? What to do? When to do?

HANDWASHING

In 1847, Dr Ignac Semmelweis, a Viennese obstetrician demonstrated that maternal mortality was very high when doctors delivered babies in hospitals when compared to deliveries conducted at home. He attributed that the increased mortality was due to infection being transferred by doctor's contaminated hands!—a finding that was later confirmed by Lister. Handwashing is the most cost-effective method of controlling healthcare-associated infections. It is a precaution, necessary prior to wearing gloves. In addition, it is preferable that healthcare providers maintain short nails to avoid the growth of microbes beneath the nails.

WHEN DO YOU WASH HANDS?

- Before touching a patient
- Before doing a procedure
- After touching a patient
- After contact with body fluids
- After touching a patient's linen or cot.

HOW TO WASH HANDS?

- Remove rings, bangles and watch.
- Moisten hands, forearm and lower third of arms with water.
- Apply soap to the arm and forearm.
- Produce a good lather.

Our hands, are colonized with organisms such as methicillin resistant S. aureus (MRSA), vancomycin resistant Enterococcus (VRE), MDR-Gram Negative bacteria (GNBs), Candida spp. and Clostridium difficle, which can survive for as long as 150 hours.

Hands, get contaminated by touching the patient's intact skin, inanimate objects in the room example: recording BP.

The WHO is currently propagating "SAVE LIVES: Clean Your Hands" program.

6 STEPS OF HANDWASHING

- Use elbow-operated or foot-operated taps to wash hands
- Wash for 40–60 seconds
- Dry hands with sterile towel or paper
- Avoid wearing gloves when the hands are wet.

In general, handwashing is recommended prior to entering into the nursery or ICU followed by hand-rub between patients. Handwash is repeated if there has been visible soiling with blood and body fluids.

If the hands are not soiled, hand-rub with an alcohol-based solution is sufficient. Duration of hand-rub is 20–30 seconds. Hand-rub takes less time and is more effective (Figures 1 to 8).

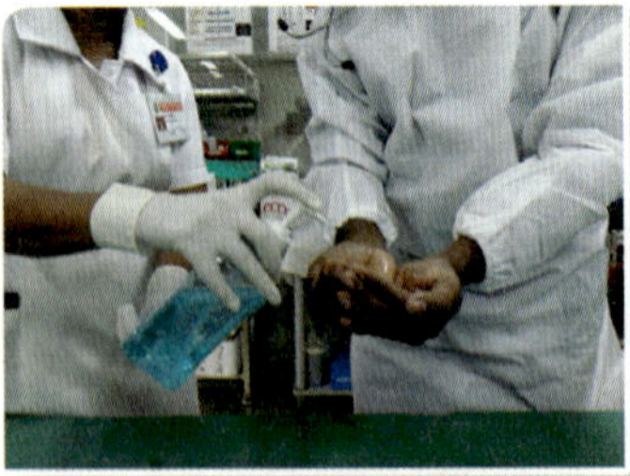

Figure 1: Take adequate hand scrub.

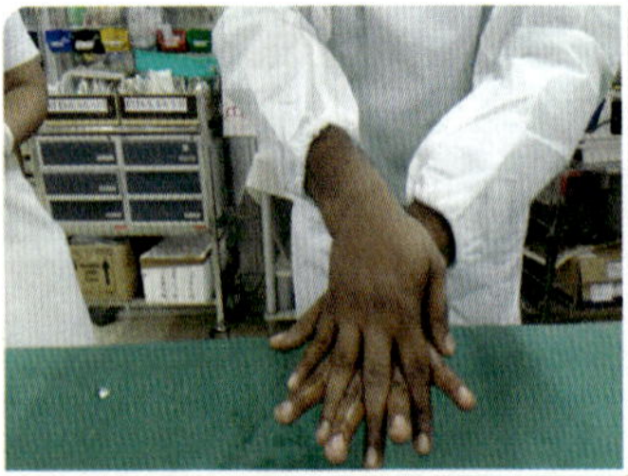

Figure 2: Rub the hand scrub palm to palm while interlacing the fingers.

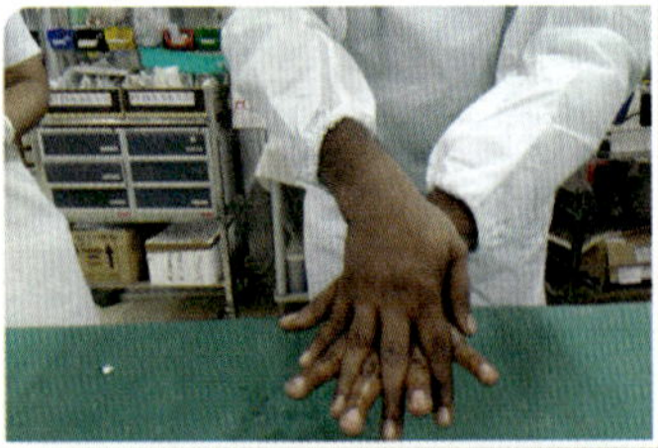

Figure 3: Right palm over left dorsum. Change hands and repeat with left palm over right dorsum.

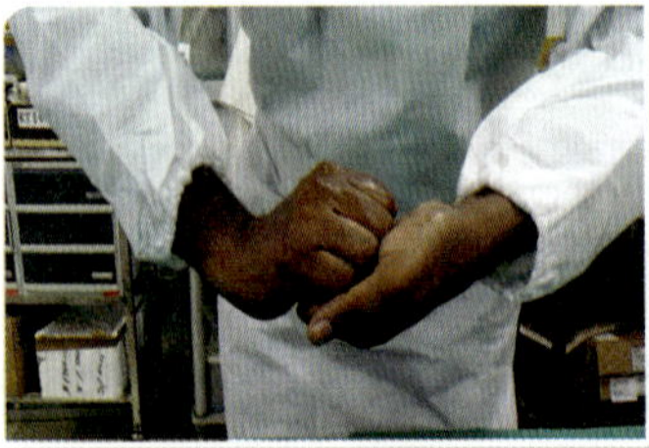

Figure 4: Back of fingers over opposing palm while inter-locking fingers.

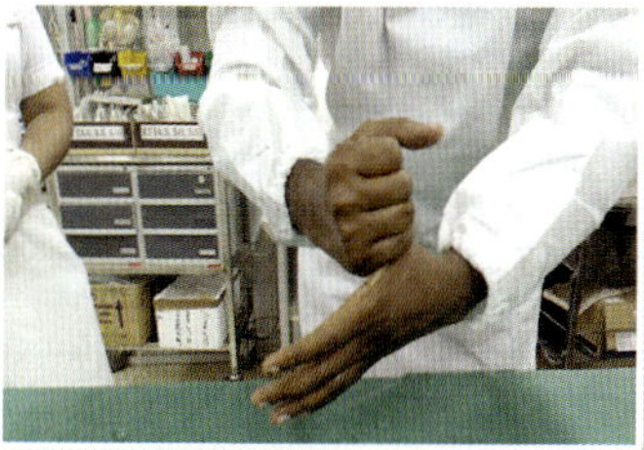

Figure 5: Rotational rubbing of right palms over left thumb.

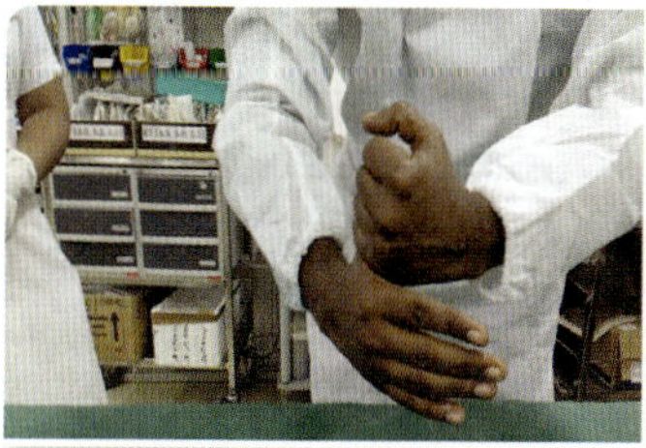

Figure 6: Change hands and repeat maneuver.

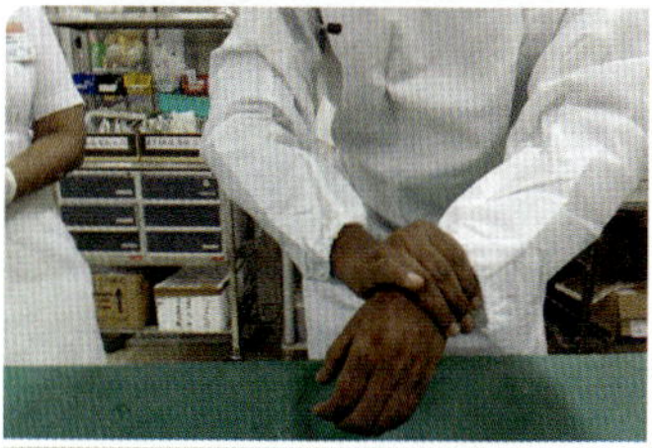

Figure 7: Rotational rub of right hand around left wrist.

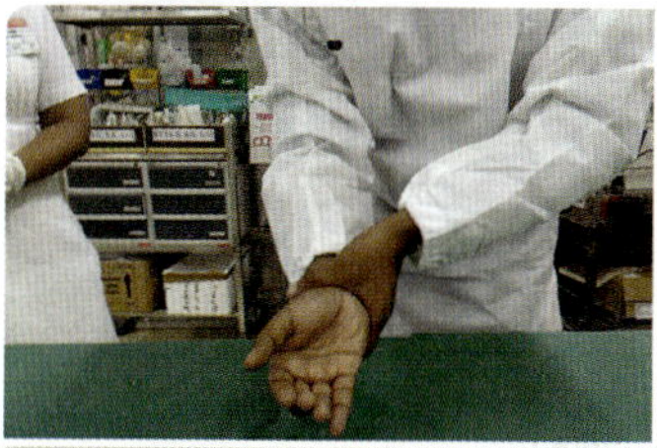

Figure 8: Change hands and repeat with the contrary hand.

WHY SHOULD YOU WEAR GLOVES?

- To protect the healthcare provider (HCP) from potentially infectious body fluids.
- To prevent spread of microorganisms from HCP to patients.

WHEN DO YOU USE STERILE GLOVES?

- Before doing any procedure.
- Prior to securing vascular access, especially a central line.
- Prior to preparing total parenteral nutrition or chemotherapeutic drugs.

WHEN DO YOU USE CLEAN GLOVES?

- Insertion or removal of a peripheral line
- Rectal examination
- Sampling blood for investigations
- Contact with mucous membranes
- Handling urine, stool and other body fluids.

HOW TO WEAR AND REMOVE GLOVES? (FIGURES 9 TO 18)

Universal Precautions (UP)

Universal precautions were initially introduced following the AIDS epidemic in 1985. This refers to the measures taken by the healthcare personnel to prevent the spread of infection between one person to another. It is based on the principle that all body fluids are potentially infectious. UP helps to prevent blood-borne diseases, such as HIV, hepatitis B and C.

Universal precautions include the following:

- Effective handwashing techniques.
- Use of personal protective equipment (PPE) to avoid contact with body fluids (blood, cerebrospinal, synovial, pleural, peritoneal, pericardial, and amniotic fluids, semen and vaginal secretions).
- Disposal of all needles and sharp objects into puncture-resistant containers.

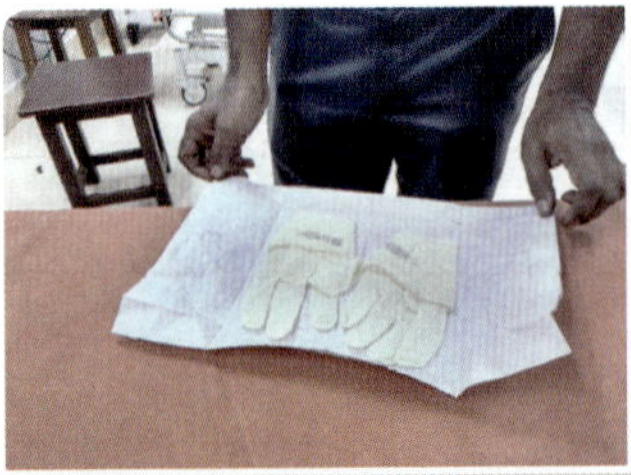

Figure 9: After washing hands as shown above, open the cover containing the gloves.

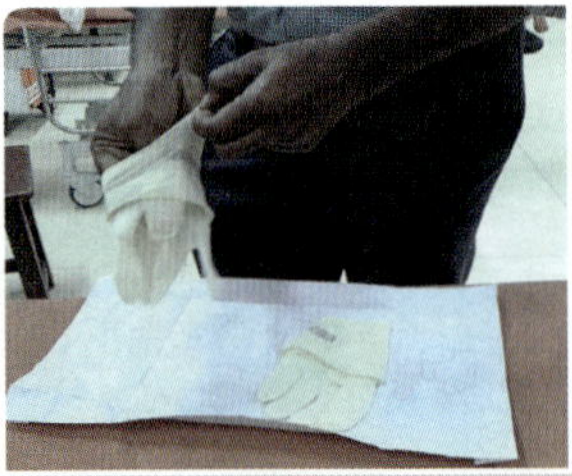

Figure 10: When wearing gloves, hook the folded end to avoid contaminating the outer surface.

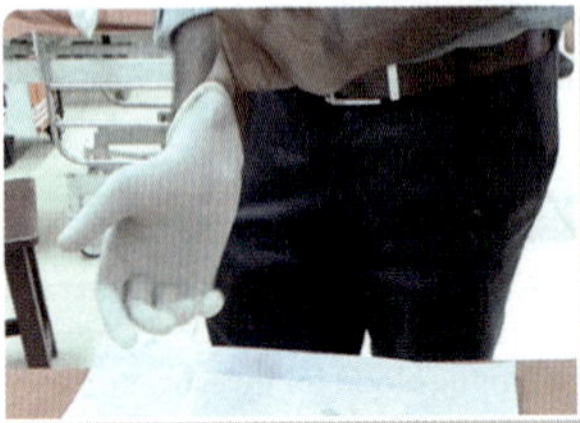

Figure 11: Pull the glove from its inner surface thereby avoid contaminating its outer surface.

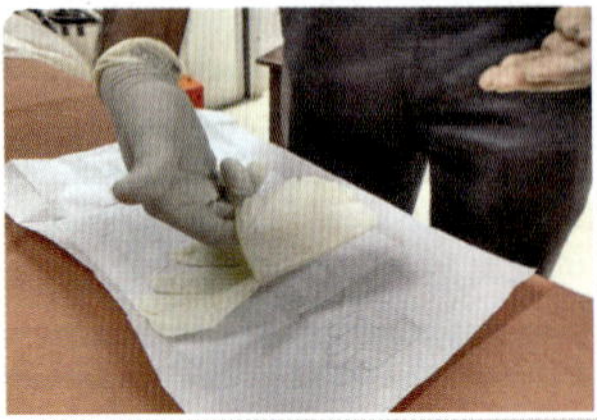

Figure 12: Use the gloved hand to insert under the folded area of the 2nd glove.

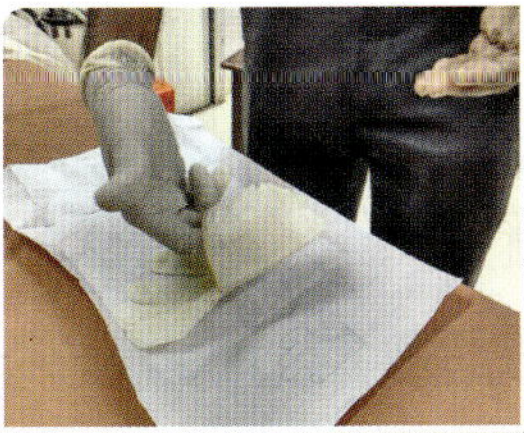

Figure 13: Use 3–4 fingers of the gloved hand to spread out the 2nd glove. This maneuver helps to insert the fingers of the 2nd hand without contaminating its surface.

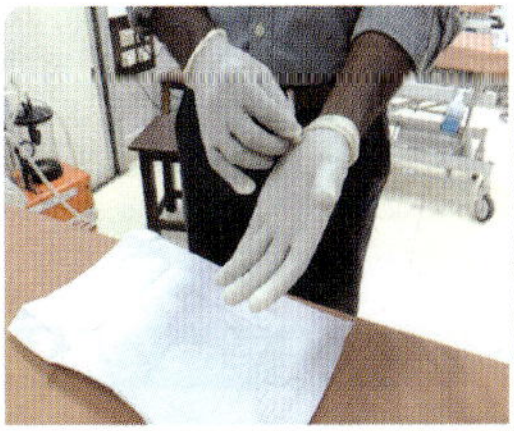

Figure 14: Ensure at all times that the gloved tip does not touch the skin.

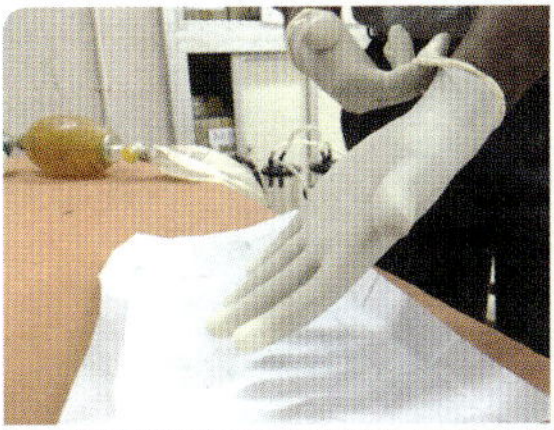

Figure 15: Removal of glove: Hook the edge of the glove at the wrist.

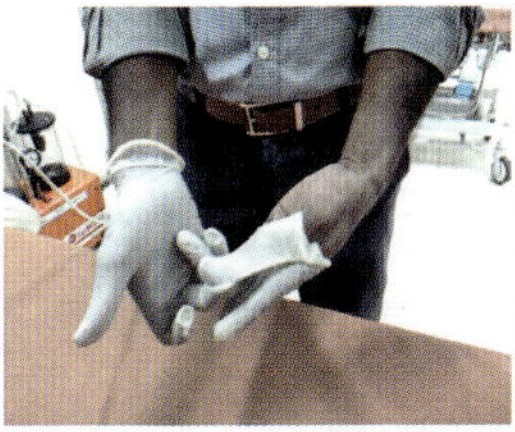

Figure 16: Peel it off without touching the used surface.

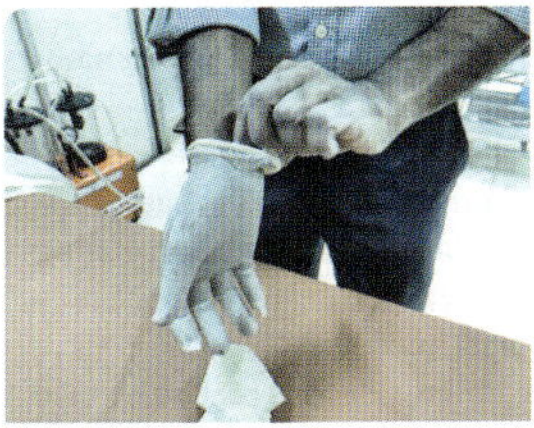

Figure 17: Hook the finger of the de-gloved hand into the inner surface of the glove at the wrist.

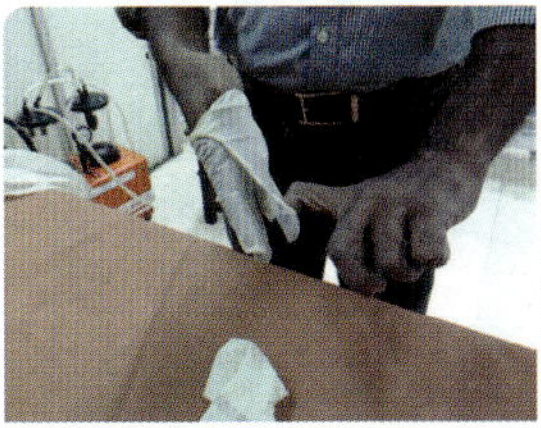

Figure 18: Peel of this glove using the hooked finger.

- Stringent precautions are taken to avoid needle-stick injury, one of which is avoidance of capping needles after use. The PPE comprises of gloves, face shield, face mask, gowns/lab coats and goggles. Gowns are worn to avoid the risk of splashing of blood or body fluids. Face mask, goggles and face shield protect against exposure of mucosa of the nose, eyes and mouth from droplets of blood or body fluid.

HOW TO DO? WHAT TO DO? WHEN TO DO?

LUMBAR PUNCTURE (FIGURES 19 TO 21)

Lumbar puncture (LP) is a procedure used to obtain samples of cerebrospinal fluid for diagnostic purposes.

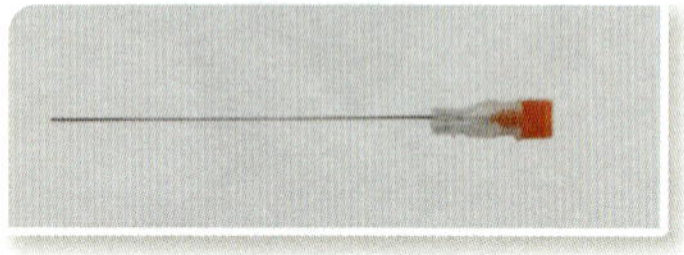

Figure 19: LP needle.

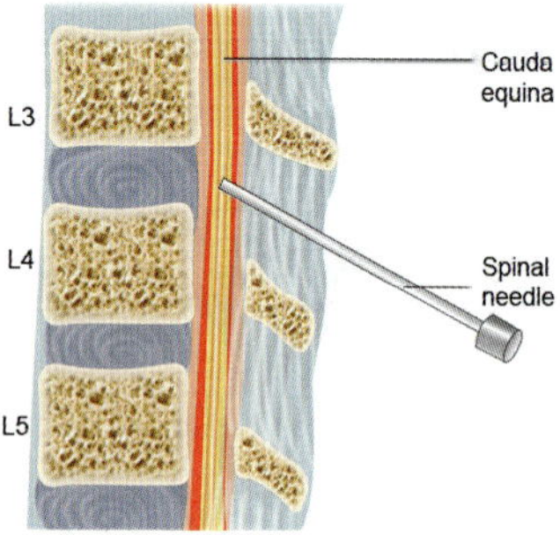

Figure 20: Lumbar puncture anatomy.

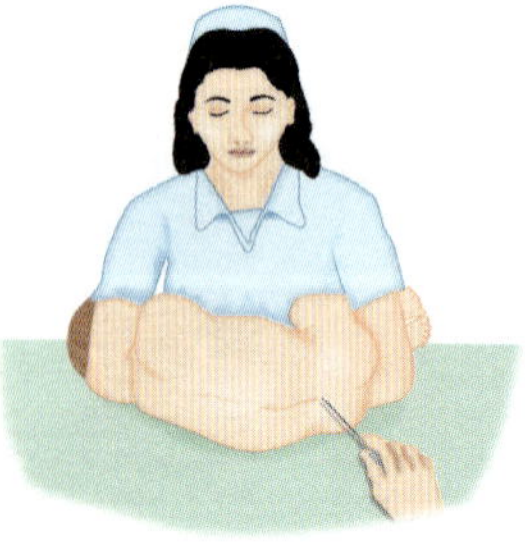

Figure 21: Positioning for a lumbar puncture.

Indications

- Meningitis (Pyogenic, Tuberculous, Viral)
- Encephalitis
- Guillain-Barre syndrome
- Subarachnoid hemorrhage
- Intrathecal administration of drugs (chemotherapy in acute leukemia)
- Spinal anesthesia
- To drain CSF in order to reduce intracranial tension. CSF drainage is therapeutic only when CT brain shows that the basal cisterns are open.

Contraindications

- Hemodynamic instability.
- Raised intracranial pressure (ICP)
- Coagulopathy
- Skin infection at the site of LP.

Precautions Taken Prior to LP

- Perform the rapid cardio-pulmonary cerebral assessment to rule out shock, cardiac dysfunction, subtle status epilepticus and raised ICP
- Fundus is examined to rule out papilledema.
- CT brain is taken to identify raised ICP (contraindication for LP).
- Patient is also examined for clinical evidence of raised ICP.
- LP is avoided if the child has features of shock or cardiac dysfunction.

Procedure

- **Informed consent is obtained prior to performing LP:**
  - The need for LP and hazards of the procedure are explained to the parents, following which written permission is taken.
- **Positioning:**
  - LP is usually performed by positioning the child in the left lateral position.
  - Place the child on a firm couch or on the bed on his or her left side such that
  - The vertebral column is parallel to this surface and the transverse axis of the back (a line passing through the posterior superior iliac spine) is vertical.
  - An assistant holds the child firmly by flexing him at the shoulders, knees and hips (Figure 21).
- **Use aseptic technique:**
  - Wash hands as described in earlier section and wear sterile gloves.
- **Method:**
  - Palpate the iliac crest. It corresponds to the fourth lumbar spine. Locate the intervertebral space between L3 and L4 or L4 and L5 vertebrae.
  - Prepare the skin around the site with an antiseptic solution (Povidone Iodine). Start from the center and proceed towards the periphery. Clean from above downwards. Drape using sterile central hole towels.
- **Pain and sedation:**
  - Ketamine is administered for pain relief and sedation [Should be administered only if (Pediatric Advanced Life Support (PALS) certified].
  - Infiltrate using local anesthetic (1% Lidocaine).
- **Procedure:**
  - Use an LP needle with stylet (22G gauge, 1.5 inches for a young infant or 20 gauge for an older infant and child); if these are not available, hypodermic needles may be used.
  - Insert the needle into the middle of the intervertebral space with the bevel pointing upwards while aiming the needle toward the umbilicus. Advance the needle slowly.

- Once the dura is penetrated and the needle is in the subarachnoid space, there will be a loss of resistance. Remove the stylet. Cerebrospinal fluid (CSF) will drip from the hollow outer end.
- Collect the fluid in 3 sterile tubes for cytology, culture and biochemical analysis. CSF pressure can be measured using a manometer.
- Once the procedure is over, introduce the stylet and withdraw the needle and stylet together.
- Apply pressure over the site for a few seconds and apply a sterile dressing over the needle puncture site. This is removed after 24 hours.

- **Documentation:**
  - The procedure is noted in the case sheet.
  - Time, complications if any and color of the sample are documented.
  - Normal CSF is colorless. Turbidity occurs due to the presence of white blood cells (WBCs) or microorganisms. Blood suggests that the procedure might have been traumatic.

Problems During LP

- If the needle has gone too far, the lumbar vein may have been punctured. This results in a "traumatic tap"! The needle should be withdrawn and the procedure repeated in another disc space, usually one space above. A traumatic tap is differentiated from a subarachnoid hemorrhage by collecting the CSF in 3 tubes.
- Improvement in the color, is suggestive that the tap is traumatic.
- Dry tap: Failure to drain CSF. This often occurs due to improper positioning of the patient.
- Post-LP headache: A slight reduction in CSF pressure, can result in severe headache. The headache resolves within 24 to 48 hours; if severe, Paracetamol can be given. Headache can be prevented by making the child lie flat for 8–24 hours after the LP.
- Some children may vomit after the LP.
- LP can lead to fatal cerebral herniation in children with ICP.

CSF Analysis

Cytology: Look for cells immediately after LP!

Normally, 0–2 lymphocytes/mL may be seen in CSF. CSF is centrifuged and the deposit is stained with Leishman's stain to study the cell characteristics. Gram's stain is performed to rule out gram-positive and gram-negative organisms. Ziehl-Neelsen stain helps recognize mycobacteria.

Biochemistry

Protein and glucose are estimated in the CSF. Normal protein is 10–40 mg/dL; Glucose is 40–80 mg/dL. CSF glucose is more than half of blood glucose. Hence, simultaneously, blood and CSF should be evaluated for glucose levels.

Microbiology

Cerebrospinal fluid is sent for culture and sensitivity for bacterial and tuberculous infection. Serological tests are performed as needed.

Common Errors

- Not examining the fundus prior to LP.
- Improper positioning of the patient.
- Not performing the rapid cardiopulmonary cerebral assessment prior to the procedure. A normal assessment, rules out hypoxia, shock, non-convulsive status epilepticus or ICP.

BONE MARROW ASPIRATION

Indications

Diagnostic

- Leukemia (diagnosis as well as immune-phenotyping)
- Aplastic anemia
- Idiopathic thrombocytopenic purpura (to exclude other causes before starting steroids)
- Marrow infiltration by:
  - Lymphoma
  - Neuroblastoma
  - Myelofibrosis
  - Storage disease (e.g. Gaucher's disease)
  - Kala-azar (LD body).

Therapeutic

- Bone marrow transplantation.
- To give resuscitation fluids in shock through the intraosseous route. Refer to Chapter on Intra-osseous Access.

Contraindications

- Local skin infection
- Hemophilia.

Parts of the Bone Marrow Needle (Figure 22)

1. Trocar (stillette) with knob
2. Cannula
3. Adjustable guard

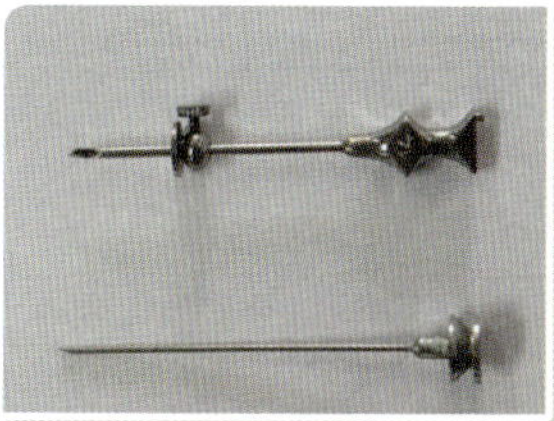

Figure 22: Bone marrow aspiration needle with trocar and cannula.

Preparation of the BM Aspiration tray:
Bone marrow aspiration needle 14.16,18 G (Figure 22)
Sterile gauze
Gamgee pad
Stainless Steel bowl-2
Straight artery forceps-2
Central hole towel -1
Towel-1
Positioning of the patient:
The child is placed in a right or left lateral decubitus position with their knees flexed, and a pillow under their head, and the eyes looking away. The posterior iliac crest is used for children over one year of age.

Site of Aspiration (Figure 23)

- Any age: Anterior and posterior superior iliac spine, iliac crest
- Birth to 2 years: Tibia—one finger breadth below and medial to the tibial tubercle on the anterior surface of the tibia. This site is often used for securing intraosseous access.

Sternum is never used in children.

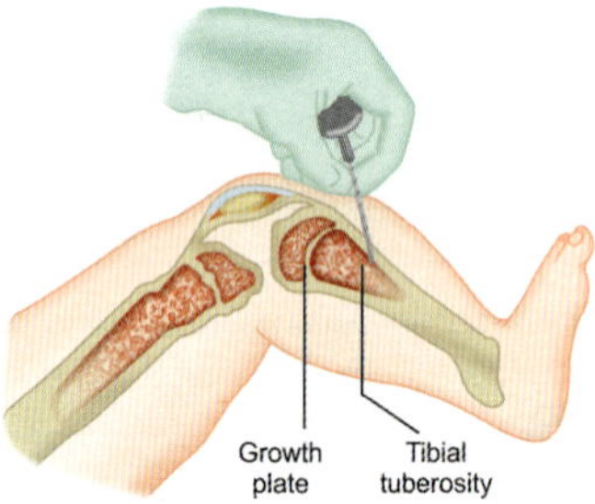

Figure 23: Bone marrow aspiration site in a young child.

Procedure

- Obtain informed consent prior to the procedure.
- Follow universal precautions.
- Fix the guard of the needle at about 1/2 the depth of bone.
- Palpate patient's back to identify anatomical landmarks.
- Mark the site of insertion by locating the dimple that corresponds to the posterior superior iliac spine.
- Prepare the site by using an antiseptic solution.
- Wear sterile gloves.
- Infiltrate local anesthetic (2% xylocaine) up to the periosteum.
- Introduce the bone marrow needle perpendicular to the skin. Once the bone is reached, use screwing motion to enter the bone.
- A sudden loss of resistance indicates that the needle has entered the marrow space. The needle will also stand straight.
- Remove the stillet and attach a 10-cc syringe to the cannula.
- Aspirate the marrow by gentle suction. Make smears.
- Withdraw the needle and apply firm pressure to the puncture site for a few minutes and then apply sterile dressing.

Complications

- Over-penetration
- Hemorrhage
- Introduction of infection (osteomyelitis)

After obtaining the marrow specimen, stop the bleed by applying pressure with thumb or fingers on to the procedure site until bleeding has completely ceased.
Clean the procedure site by disposing, needles in a sharps container.
Bandage the site.
Document the procedure in the child's chart.

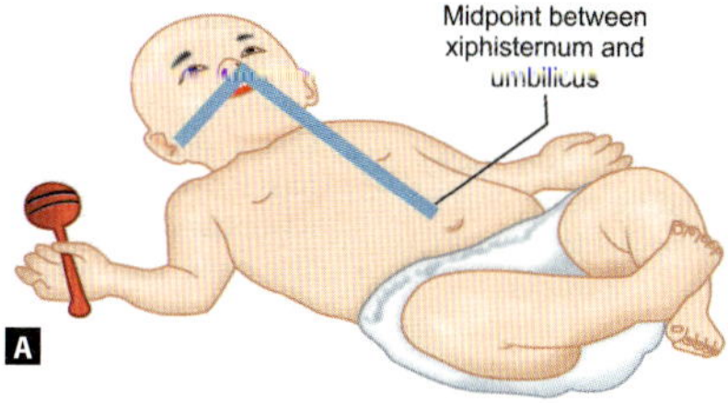

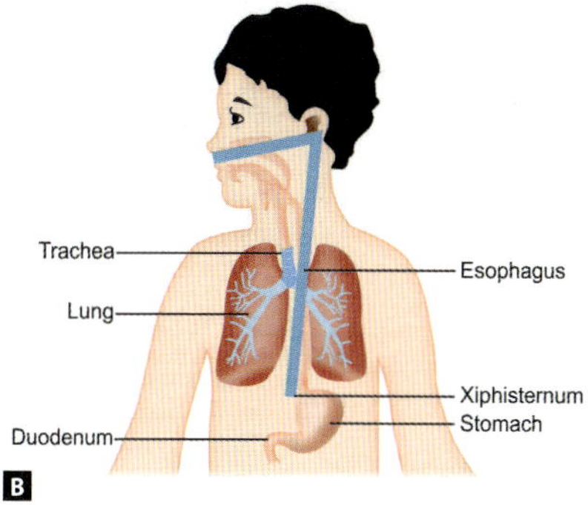

Figures 24A and B: Measuring an NG tube (A) for an infant; (B) for a child.

NASOGASTRIC TUBE INSERTION (FIGURES 24A AND B)

A nasogastric tube (NGT) is a narrow bore tube passed into the stomach via the nose.

Indications

- Short- or medium-term nutritional support.
- Aspiration of stomach contents and decompression of stomach before bag mask ventilation.
- Stomach wash in children who have ingested toxin.
- The nasogastric tube is radiopaque throughout its length with visible markings.
- Diagnose tracheoesophageal fistula in the neonate.
- Collection of resting gastric juice for testing for acid-fast bacilli.

Contraindications

Upper gastrointestinal stricture, nasal injuries and base of skull fractures.

Types of NGT

The NGTs are radiopaque throughout their length and have externally visible markings. The range extends from 5 Fr to 10 Fr. Polyurethane or silicone-feeding tubes can be used up to 30 days. Polyvinyl chloride (PVC) tubes can only be used for 1–2 weeks.

Equipment Needed

1. Nasogastric tube of appropriate size
2. 5 mL syringe
3. Lubricant (sterile water or water- soluble lubricants)
4. Stethoscope
5. Suction equipment
6. Plaster

Procedure

- Obtain informed consent.
- Place the young child in the supine position with the neck mildly extended such that the nose is pointing upward. Placing a rolled towel under the neck will facilitate this position. The older child can be seated.
- Ask the parent or another person to hold the child.
- Wash your hands, dry and wear clean gloves.
- Select the age-appropriate-sized tube.
- Measure the length of tube to be inserted. It is estimated by measuring the distance from the tip of the nose to the ear lobe and from the ear lobe to the xiphisternum.
- In the neonate, it is measured from the tip of the nose to the ear lobe and from the earlobe to a point midway between the xiphisternum and the umbilicus. Hold the tube at the measured point and lubricate the tube liberally with sterile water or water soluble.
- Gently pass the tube into the nostril. Direct the tube slightly upwards and pass it over the back of the nose into the nasopharynx.
- The child may gag or vomit when the tube reaches the back of the throat. Ask the older child to swallow. Advance the tube as the child swallows till the required length is introduced.

Remove the NGT if the child develops respiratory distress, cyanosis or gasping as these signs indicate that the tube has entered the trachea.

Check Tube Position

1. Aspiration of gastric contents. The color of the aspirate may be clear, tan, green, bloody, brown or cloudy.
2. Inject 5 mL of air into the NGT with a syringe and place the stethoscope in the epigastric region and listen "Whoosh test".

Although this is the most commonly performed, this test is not supported by recent evidence.

3. Take an X-ray to check the position of the tube in the stomach. This is confirmatory.
4. Check pH using pH indicator strip. Do not use litmus paper. If pH is < 6, it indicates appropriate tube placement.

Fixing

- After confirmation of tube position, secure the tube to the skin with plaster and flush the tube with water.

Documentation

- Document the date and time, as well as the size and type of tube that has been used. Record the length of tube that has been inserted, the length of visible tube from the nostril to the end (i.e. outside the child's body) and record that correct placement has been confirmed.

Maintenance of NGT

- The NGT can easily get displaced when the child coughs or vomits. Hence, check tube position before feeding or administering drugs and at least once daily if continuous feeds are given to prevent aspiration.
- Flush the NGT with water after administering medications or feeds.
- Children may pull out the tubes and re-insertion is frequently needed.

Complications

- Tracheal insertion
- Perforation
- Aspiration of gastric contents
- Gastroesophageal reflux if tube is kept for a longer period
- Injury to the nose and damage to the skin on the face.

Common Errors

1. Not measuring the length of the tube to be inserted.
2. Not checking the position of the NGT before giving feeds or medications.
3. Not lubricating the NGT before insertion.

Urethral Catheterization (Figures 25A to C)

Strict asepsis is essential for urethral catheterization. UTI in turn, can cause renal scar-

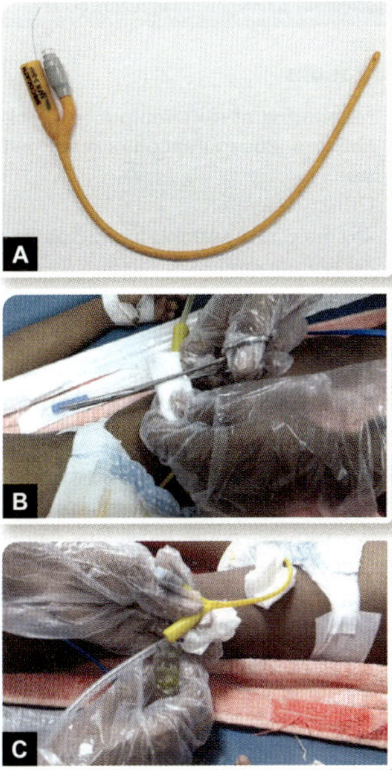

Figures 25A to C: (A) Foley's catheter; (B) Clamp, foley's catheter with an artery forceps prior to disconnection. Release to collect sample; (C) Release the clamp and collect urine in a sterile manner. Additionally observe universal precautions.

ring, chronic renal failure or hypertension in later life. Hence, catheterization is performed only when absolutely indicated.

Introduction of microorganisms into the urinary tract during catheterization can cause iatrogenic urinary tract infection (UTI).

Indications

- Monitoring of urine output in shocked children aids evaluation of renal perfusion.
- Urinary retention.
- To collect urine sample for microbiological examination.
- Neurogenic bladder.

Contraindication

Pelvic fracture with suspected urethral injury.

PARTS OF THE FOLEY'S TUBE (FIGURE 25A)

Foley's catheter is the indwelling catheter used in children. It consists of two lumens; one for an inflatable balloon and the other a conduit for urine. A feeding tube is used for neonates and young infants. A rough guide for selecting the size of the tube is given below.

- 6F (French gauge) for infants; 8F for toddlers and early school age; 10F for older children and adolescents.

Avoid

- Use of a larger size for the age will cause painful spasm, bleeding, blockage of urethral glands and ulceration of bladder neck.

Equipment Needed

- Alcohol hand rub
- 2 sterile gloves
- Appropriately sized Foley's catheter
- Lignocaine jelly
- Sterile syringes
- Sterile towels
- Antiseptic solution (povidone iodine)
- Sterile bowl
- Sterile gauze swabs
- Sterile tubes to collect urine
- Adhesive tapes
- Plastic apron.

Procedure

- Get informed consent.
- Ask for history of allergy to latex.
- Ensure privacy.
- Clean the genital area with soap and water if there is soiling.
- Wash your hands. Dry. Use alcohol rub.
- Plastic apron is worn to prevent splash.
- Wear sterile gloves.
- Set the tray ready. Pour antiseptic in a cup. Keep the syringe filled up with water to inflate the balloon. Open the cover of the Foley's catheter and keep it ready.
- Position the child supine with the legs slightly apart.
- Clean the perineal and genital area, the inner aspects of the thigh and the lower aspect of the abdomen up to the umbilicus with antiseptic solution and apply sterile drapes beneath the child's thighs and over the abdomen.

- Boys: Hold the penis with a gauze using the non-dominant hand and with the other hand, clean the glans penis with a sterile gauze soaked in antiseptic solution. Do not retract the prepuce fully.
- Girls: Separate the labia with one hand and (Figure 26) with the other hand, clean the area from front to back with a sterile gauze soaked in antiseptic solution and discard it. Use a new sterile gauze for each stroke.

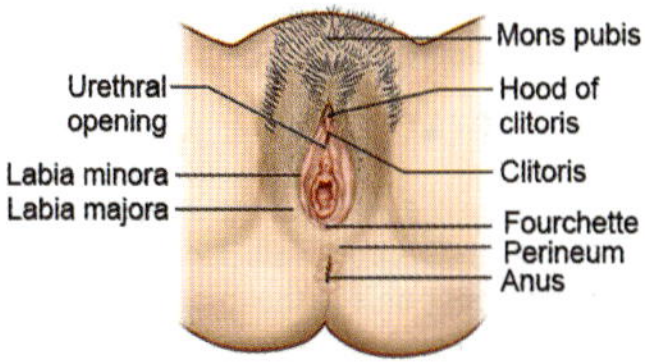

Figure 26: Position of urethra in the girl child

- Apply lignocaine gel into the urethral meatus and wait for a few minutes to act.
- Remove the glove and wear a new sterile glove.
- Introduce the catheter gently into the meatus with the end to be connected to the urine collecting bag still within the plastic cover. Do not use force.
- Ensure that the tip of the catheter does not touch the skin or surrounding area to prevent contamination with microorganisms.
- Once the catheter enters the bladder, urine flows out. Advance the catheter to 2–4 cm. Remove the plastic cover.
- Collect urine in sterile tubes, if needed, for investigations.
- Inject sterile water (Figures 25B and C) to inflate the bulb (the quantity as per the specifications of the manufacturer). This helps the catheter remain in place.
- Withdraw the catheter slightly till mild resistance is felt.
- Reposition foreskin (in boys, if retracted).
- Connect the other end to the urine collecting bag. The bag should always be at a level lower than the bladder. It is usually tied to the side of the cot. Make sure the bag does not touch the floor.
- Fix the catheter onto the thigh or abdomen. Ensure there is a loop in the catheter while fixing to prevent traction on the urethra when the child moves.
- Document the procedure in the child's medical record. Documentation should include indication for catheterization, time and date of procedure, type and size of catheter, amount of water in balloon, problems during insertion, description of urine, color and volume, investigations sent. The documentation should be signed by the person inserting the catheter.

Complications

- Urethral trauma
- Hematuria
- Urethral stricture
- Infection
- Paraphimosis in boys if prepuce is not repositioned.

If catheter is not draining urine, it is examined for kinks, displacement, blockage, and leak. The most common cause of failure to drain is a block in the catheter.

Common Errors

- Not using double gloves.
- Complete retraction of the prepuce and failing to reposition it after the procedure is complete.

Suprapubic Aspiration of Urine (Figure 27)

Indications

- To obtain uncontaminated urine for microbiology.

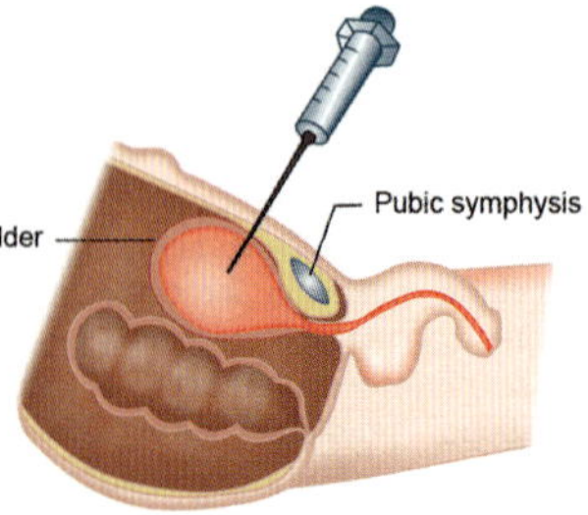

Figure 27: Suprapubic aspiration of urine.

Equipment Required

- Antibacterial solution, e.g. chlorhexidine or povidone iodine
- Sterile dressing pack
- 22G (blue) needle
- 10 mL syringe
- Container.

Position

- Place the infant in the supine position. An assistant or parent firmly holds the legs in position.
- Confirm whether the bladder is full either by palpation or ultrasound.
- Ensure that a container is available to obtain a clean catch sample. Spontaneous urination is not uncommon during the procedure.

Use Strict Aseptic Precautions

- Clean the skin of lower abdomen with antibacterial solution.
- Use an alcohol swab.

Procedure

- Insert needle with syringe attached at 90° to the abdominal wall, 1 cm above the symphysis pubis in the midline.
- Advance needle slowly to depth of 1–2 cm, while aspirating continuously until urine is obtained.
- Aspirate as much urine as possible and send for microbiology (culture and sensitivity).
- Remove needle and apply pressure to puncture site.

Complications

- Bladder trauma and hematuria
- Bowel puncture.

PERIPHERAL VEIN CANNULATION (FIGURES 28 TO 30)

Starting an intravenous line in children may be difficult, but the technique can be mastered by constant practice.

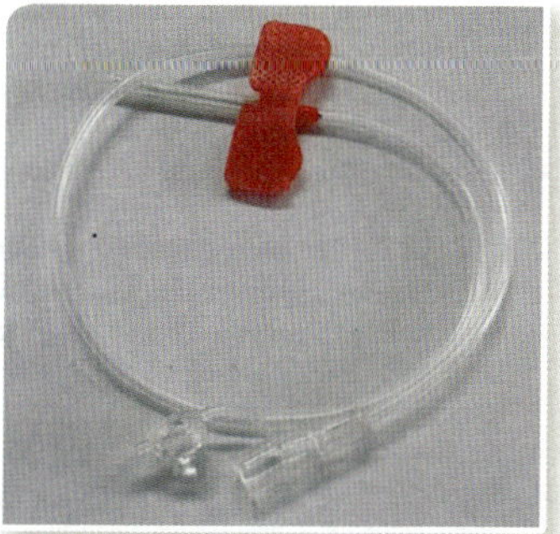

Figure 28: Butterfly needle. More useful to collect blood sample.

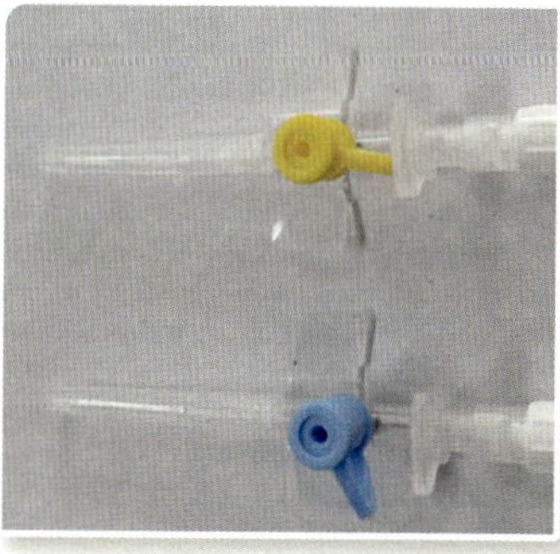

Figure 29: Over-the-needle catheters.

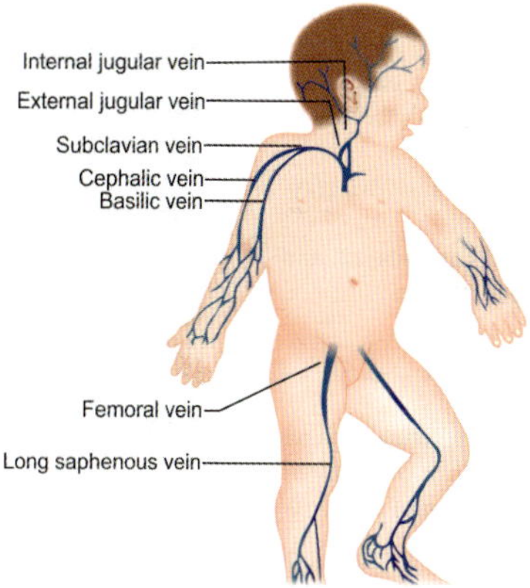

Figure 30: Common veins used for intravenous infusion or sampling in infants.

The commonly used peripheral veins are veins of the dorsal venous arch in the hands or feet, the cephalic and the basilic veins of the lower arm, the saphenous vein or sometimes the scalp vein. In an emergency, the veins in the antecubital fossa (median cubital vein) and external jugular veins are used. Avoid areas of flexion except in an emergency. Avoid previously punctured or thrombosed veins. Choose a vein which is visible, easy to palpate and has a straight course preferably on the non-dominant hand.

Devices Used

- Butterfly needles—useful for scalp veins. It is also used for venipuncture to collect blood for investigations.
- Over-the-needle catheters—commonly known as intravenous (IV) cannula. These are most commonly employed. There are different sizes for different age groups and are color- coded.
  Yellow-24G; blue-22G; purple-20G; gray-18G; green-16G;
  22 and 24G are used for infants. 22, and 20G are used for older children.

Procedure

- Obtain informed consent.
- Apply topical local anesthetics such as Eutectic Mixture of Local Anesthetic (EMLA) cream one hour prior to the IV insertion (elective IV access).
- Ensure adequate lighting.
- Follow universal precautions.
- Immobilize the extremity to be used and identify the appropriate vein.
- Ask an assistant to hold the limb proximal to the vein. This makes the vein more prominent. For older children, apply a tourniquet proximal to the vein.
- Keep bottles/tubes ready to collect blood for investigations.
- 5 mL of 0.9 normal saline in a syringe ready to flush and check proper position.
- Syringe, filled with saline is kept ready to flush and check position of the IV cannula.
- Wash hands and put on gloves.
- Clean the skin over the vein with an antiseptic solution, either povidone iodine or 2% chlorhexidine in 70% alcohol. Allow it to dry for 30 seconds. Once cleaned, skin should not be re-palpated (Figures 31A and B).

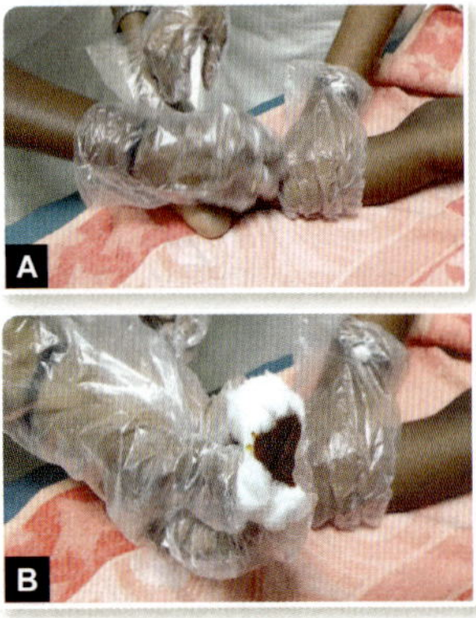

Figures 31A and B: (A) After cleaning avoid touching the skin in order to palpate the vein, (B) clean with povidone iodine and allow to dry for 30 seconds.

- Choose the appropriate sized cannula.
- Stretch the skin below the insertion to anchor the vein. Insert over-the-needle catheter into the vein (Figure 32) at an appropriate angle with bevel of the needle facing upward.

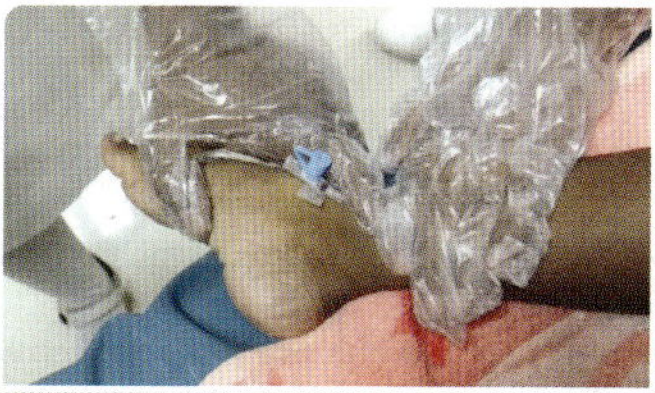

Figure 32: Once blood is seen at the hub, the needle is withdrawn and the cannula is inserted.

- Once the needle is in the vein, the blood flows back freely. Advance the catheter a few millimeters further to ensure that the catheter is in the vein. Advance the remainder of the catheter over the needle and into the vein till the hub.
- Remove the needle. Apply pressure over the vein above the cannula while removing the needle (Figure 33).

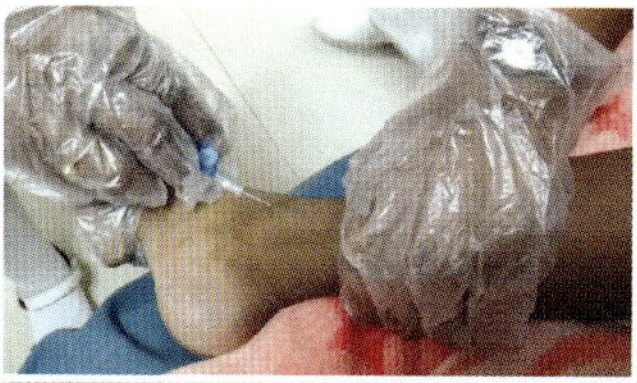

Figure 33: Stretch the skin prior to insertion of venflon.

- Collect blood for investigations if needed.
- Connect the syringe filled with normal saline and flush to make sure there is no extravasation (Figure 34).

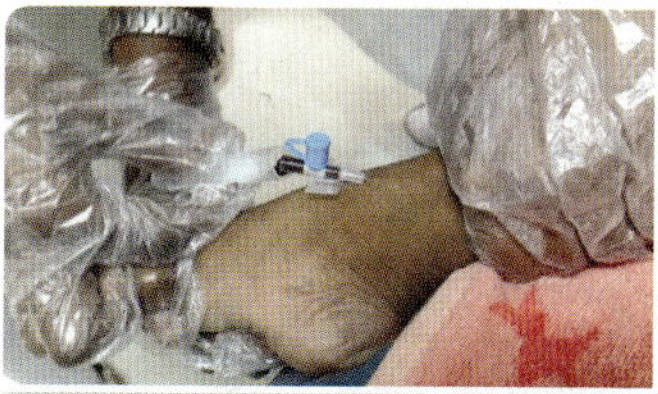

Figure 34: In severe shock, it may not be possible to collect blood. In which case, prioritize fluid resuscitation.

Prior to securing IV access, prepare an IV infusion by connecting the IV set to the reservoir. Ensure that the IV set tip is closed until it is connected.

- Remove the tourniquet if applied earlier.
- Secure the cannula with plaster.
- Attach an infusion set after letting out air in the tubing (Figure 35).

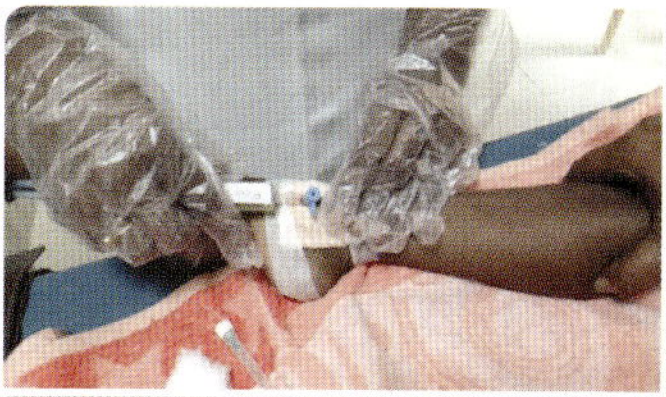

Figure 35: Secure the venflon with dynaplast.

- Immobilize the limb with a splint in young infants.
- Remove gloves and wash hands.
- Dispose sharps and all equipment appropriately.

Complications

- Hematoma formation
- Cellulitis
- Infection
- Extravasation
- Infiltration of drugs
- Thrombophlebitis
- Skin slough
- Pain
- Rarely pulmonary thromboembolism, air embolism and catheter fragment embolism
- Needle stick injuries or sharp injuries.

Caution

Certain drugs, such as dopamine, epinephrine, calcium can cause vasculitis. These drugs should be diluted and administered through the largest veins. Infusion site should be closely monitored. When in doubt or the child complains of pain, stop the infusion, remove the line and start a new one.

Common Errors

- Palpating the vein after cleaning with antiseptic.
- Touching the hub of the cannula with cotton to stop bleeding.
- Placing the syringe or IV infusion set on patient's bed without cap.
- Not wearing gloves while starting an IV line.

14

CHAPTER

Clinical Aids

Chapter Outline

- Drug Dosage and Indications in Children
- Appendices

ANTIBIOTICS

I.	**Aminoglycosides**	
	Indication	UTI, Intra-abdominal infections, Sepsis and Gram negative infections
	Side effect	Renal toxicity and ototoxicity
	1. Amikacin	15–25 mg/kg/day bd or tds
	2. Gentamicin	2.5 mg/kg/dose 8–12 hrly
II.	**Penicillin**	
1.	Phenoxymethyl penicillin (Penicillin V)	25–50 mg/kg/day 6–8 hrly
	Acute group A Streptococcal pharyngitis	250–500 mg/dose (bd-tds x 10 days)
	Rheumatic fever prophylaxis	< 5 yrs => 125 mg/dose bd po > 5 yrs => 250 mg/dose bd po
2.	Ampicillin	50–300 mg/kg/day IV in 4 divided doses for mild-to-serious infection
3.	Amoxycillin	25–40 mg/kg/day in 2–3 divided doses up to 80 mg/kg/day in severe infections like otitis media
4.	Amoxycillin with clavulanic acid	Dosage based upon amoxycillin component
	Side effect	Diarrhea and measles-like rash of Piperacillin component
5.	Piperacillin + tazobactam	200–300 mg/kg/day 6–8 hrly
6.	Betalactamine-resistant Penicillin: Cloxacillin	Children: 50–100 mg/kg/day in 4 divided doses (1–2 hrs before meals) 25 mg/kg/day in newborn Mainly for S. aureus infections Skin and soft-tissue infections

Contd...

Contd...

	Side effects	Nausea, rash, eosinophilia, diarrhea
III.	**Macrolides**	
1.	Erythromycin	20-30 mg/kg/day in 3-4 divided doses
	Contraindications	Simultaneous use with Terfenadine, Osterizole with Cisapride causes cardiac arrhythmias
	Side effects	Nausea, vomiting and cholestatic jaundice
2.	Azithromycin	i. > 6 months => 10 mg/kg/dose o.d. for 3 days (OR) ii. 10 mg/kg/dose for day 1 for 5 mg/kg/day × 4 days iii. 20 mg/kg/day o.d. for Enteric fever 1 hr before (or) 2 hrs after meals
3.	Clarithromycin	15 mg/kg/day 12 hrly
4.	Clindamycin	10–25 mg/kg/day in 4 divided doses (covers Staph. and Anaerobes)
	Side effects	Diarrhoea, pseudomembranous colitis
IV.	**Cephalosporins**	
1.	Cephalexin	25–50 mg/kg/24 hrs in 3 or 4 divided doses oral
2.	Cefadroxil	30 mg/kg/24 hrs in 2 divided doses (O)
3.	Cefazolin	50–100 mg/kg/24 hrs Q-8 hrs
4.	Cefaclor	20–40 mg/kg/24 hrs in 3 divided doses
5.	Cefuroxime Axetil	30 mg/kg/24 hrs Q-12 hrs
6.	Cefprozil	30 mg/kg/day in 2 divided doses
7.	Cefixime	10–15 mg/kg/24 hrs – 12th hrly 20 mg/kg/day (Enteric fever)
8.	Cefdinir	14 mg/kg/day – 12th hrly
9.	Cefotaxime	100–200 mg/kg/day – tds
10.	Ceftriaxone	50–75 mg/kg/day in 2 divided doses IV. 80–100 mg/kg/day in 2 divided doses IV in Meningitis. Max-4 gm/day.
11.	Cefpodoxime	10 mg/kg/day – b.d oral.
V.	**Nitrofurans**	
1.	Nitrofurantoin	5–7 mg/kg/day – t.d.s. or q.i.d. UTI prophylaxis: 1–2.5 mg/kg/day HS PO
	Side effects	Avoid in infants <3 months, G6 PD deficiency, Renal insufficiency.

Contd...

Contd...

VI.	**Sulfonamides**	
1.	Cotrimoxazole Trimethoprim-sulfamethoxazole	Dosage based on trimethoprim component 8 mg trimethoprim/day – b.i.d.
	Side effect	Hemolytic anemia in G6PD deficiency, Stevens-Johnson syndrome
VII.	**Fluoroquinolones**	
	Mainly used for Dysentery, UTI, Enteric fever and Neonatal sepsis No absolute contraindications in children	
1.	Ciprofloxacin	
	Side effects	Epigastric distress, seizures
		PO: 20–30 mg/kg/day b.d. IV: 10–20 mg/kg/day b.d.
		Do not administer antacids with oral ciprofloxacin
2.	Ofloxacin	10 mg/kg/day b.d.
3.	Norfloxacin	6–12 mg/kg/day b.d. od or bd
4.	Levofloxacin	5–10 mg/kg/dose
VIII.	**Metronidazole**	
1.	Metronidazole	30-50mg/kg/day in 3 divided doses Oral. 7.5 mg/kg/dose every 8th hrly IV as infusion. Indications: Amoebiasis in elderly child, Giardiasis, Trichomoniasis, Anaerobic infection, Pseudomembranous colitis
	Side effects	Nausea, vomiting, metallic taste
IX.	**Oxazolidinones**	
1.	Linezolid	10 mg/kg/dose b.d. oral and IV Good oral bio-availability LRI, skin and soft tissue infection and Gram +ve sepsis Mainly used for resistant gram +ve organisms, like Streptococcus, Staph. aureus, Pneumococci, Enterococcus and Listeria
X.	**Tetracyclines**	
1.	Tetracycline	25–50 mg/kg/day–6 hrs 1 hr before (or) 2 hrs after meals
2.	Doxycycline	2–5 mg/kg/day Mainly used for Cholera and Scrub typhus. May be used < 8 years also
	Side effects	GI upset, teeth-staining

Contd...

Contd...

XI.	**Chloramphenicol**	
	Chloramphenicol	50–100 mg/kg/day 6th hourly IV/PO
	Side effect	Bone marrow suppression, aplastic anemia

MALARIA TREATMENT—NEW GUIDELINES

	Uncomplicated	Complicated
Falciparum	Artesunate combination therapy* ACT-SP Artesunate (50 mg tab) 4 mg/kg for 3 days Sulfadoxine (500 mg) 25 mg/kg for 1st day Pyrimethamine (25 mg) 1.25 mg/kg alone	Artesunate IV or IM # < 20 kg–3 mg/kg >20 kg–2.4 mg/kg Or quinine or artemether** Artemether 3.2 mg/kg IM followed by 1.6 mg/kg IM daily Quinine (IM) 20 mg salt/kg initially 10 mg/kg 8 hrly, until improvement After 48 hrs, 10 mg/kg every 12 hrs
Falciparum	Give primaquine 0.75 mg/kg single dose on Day 2	
Other species (vivax, ovale, malaria, knowlesi)	Chloroquine – sensitive D1 10 mg/kg D2 10 mg/kg D3 5 mg/kg + Primaquine 0.25 mg/kg × 14 days (vivax , ovale – 14 days) Malariae – 0.75 mg/kg – single dose) Chloroquine-resistant areas—ACT	Same as for falciparum

*ACT—AL Artemether Lumefantrine in north-eastern states

* Alternatives for ACT:

1. Artesunate + clinda/doxy
2. Quinine + clinda
3. Quinine + doxy

*Available ACT

1. ASP
2. ACT—AL
3. Artesunate + amodiaquine
4. Artesunate + lumefantrine
5. Dihydroartemisinin + piperaquine

Once patient has received atleast 24 hrs of parenteral therapy and can tolerate oral therapy, complete treatment with 3 days of an ACT.
** If parenteral artesunate is not available, use IM artemether in preference to quinine for treating severe malaria.
*** PRE-REFERRAL treatment: If IM artesunate not available, treat children < 6 yrs with single rectal dose 10 mg/kg of artesunate and refer immediately.
*Mixed infections: ACT × 3 days + Primaquine 0.25 mg/kg × 14 days

ANTHELMINTICS

1.	**Albendazole**	More than 2 years: 400 mg—single dose 1–2 years: 200 mg—single dose
2.	**Mebendazole**	100 mg bd for 3 days
	Indications	Ascariasis, ankylostomiasis, trichuriasis and strongyloidiasis. Repeat after 3 weeks
3.	**Ivermectin**	0.2 mg/kg single dose
	Indications	**Scabies**, pediculosis, ascariasis, cutaneous larva migrans, strongyloidiasis

ANTI-VIRAL THERAPY

1.	**Acyclovir**	80 mg/kg/day – 4 to 5 times a day oral 30 mg/kg/day – t.d.s. IV
	Indications	Chickenpox, Herpes simplex
2.	**Oseltamivir**	<15 kg: 30 mg b.d. 2 weeks-1 year : 3 mg/kg/dose b.d 15–23 kg: 45 mg b.d. 23–40 kg: 60 mg b.d. > 40 kg: 75 mg b.d.
	Indications	Swine flu (H1N1)

ANTI-FUNGAL

1.	**Ketoconazole**	3 mg/kg/dose b.i.d.
2.	**Fluconazole**	Oropharyngeal Candidiasis: 6 mg/kg stat after 24 hrs; 3 mg/kg PO for 7 days Severe infections: 12 mg/kg stat, then 6 mg/kg/day for 7–14 days IV PO

AVOID FIXED DOSE ANTIBIOTIC COMBINATIONS

Combinations of quinolones with anti-parasitic drugs
(Norflox and metronidazole/Oflox and metronidazole/Oflox and nitazoxanide)

ANTI-EMETICS

1.	**Domperidone**	0.2–0.4 mg/kg/dose 8th hrly
2.	**Ondansetron**	Oral/IV – 0.1–0.2 mg/kg/dose 6-12 hrly
3.	**Metoclopramide**	0.1–0.3 mg/kg/dose 8th hrly (IV, IM, Oral)
	Side effects of Metoclopramide	Extrapyramidal reaction
	Antidotes	1. Diphenhydramine (Benadryl) 5 mg/kg/day (3 to 4 divided doses)
		2. Diazepam

ANTI-HISTAMINICS

Use only if allergic symptoms are noted: Sneezing, itching.

1.	**Chlorpheniramine maleate**	0.35 mg/kg/day in 4 divided doses
2.	**Pheniramine maleate (Avil)**	1.5 mg/kg/day 8 hrly
3.	**Promethazine HCL (Phenergan)**	0.5 mg/kg/dose (night) 0.1 mg/kg/dose 6 hrly
	Vomiting	0.5 mg/kg/dose 4–6 hrly
	Sedation	0.5–1 mg/kg/doe 6 hrly
	Motion sickness	0.5 mg/kg/dose – 30–60 mts before departure
4.	**Cetirizine**	2.5–5 mg/day 2–6 years 5–10 mg/day 6–12 years
5.	**Levocetirizine**	6–11 years => 2.5 mg/od > 12 years => 5 mg/od
6.	**Hydroxyzine (Atarax)**	2 mg/kg/dose 8 hrly Mainly for skin allergies like urticaria

ANTI-PEPTIC ACID DRUGS

1.	**Ranitidine**	IV => 1 mg/kg/dose 6-8 hrly Oral => 2–4 mg/kg/dose 12 hrly
2.	**Omeprazole**	0.4-0.8 mg/kg/day 1–2 divided doses
3.	**Lanzoprazole**	1.5 mg/kg/day Max. 30 mg
4.	**Sucralfate**	10–20 mg/kg/dose 4 times/day

ANTI-ASTHMA DRUGS

1.	**Adrenaline**	0.01 ml/kg of 1 in 1000 solution Subcutaneous for near fatal asthma Max single dose – 0.3 ml Repeat every 20 min for 3 doses
		Nebulization of Adrenaline helpful in ALTB (Croup) and Bronchiolitis
2.	**Ipratropium bromide**	Nebulization: 1 ml every 6–8 hrly
	Nebulizer Respirator Solution	=> 0.25 mg/2 ml
	Respule	=> 0.5 mg/2 ml
	Side effects	Dry mouth, blurred vision, urinary retention and epistaxis
3.	**Salbutamol**	Oral: 0.1–0.15 mg/kg/dose 8 hrly Nebulizer solution: (5 mg/ml) 0.15 mg/kg/dose (0.03 ml/kg/dose)
	Total volume in Nebulizer chamber	=> 3 to 4 ml
	Hypoxic asthmatics	=> Nebulize with O_2
	Avoid in wheeze not due to asthma	Salbutamol nebulization contraindicated as it can cause VP mismatch and worsen the situation
4.	**Terbutaline**	PO: 0.05 mg/kg/dose 8 hrly SC: 0.005–0.01 mg/kg/dose
	Nebulization	0.01–0.03 mg/kg
	Beta-2 Adrenergic Agonist side effects	Tachycardia, flushing, headache, tremor, dry throat, hypokalemia
5.	**Theophylline**	6 months–1 yr => 12–18 mg/kg/day every 6 hours 1–9 y => 20–25 mg/kg/day 9–12 y => 15 mg/kg/day
	Side effects	Tachycardia, irritability, arrhythmia, seizures
6.	**Budesonide**	Nebulization: 0.25–0.5 mg twice a day
	Side effect	Oropharyngeal candidiasis, epistaxis
7.	**Prednisolone**	1–2 mg/kg/day in 3 divided doses

Contd...

Contd...

8.	**Hydrocortisone**	10 mg/kg IV Stat followed by 5 mg/kg/dose 6 hrly
9.	**Dexamethasone**	0.2 mg/kg/dose 6 hrly
10.	**Betamethasone**	0.2 mg/kg/day 8 hrly
11.	**Montelukast**	For asthma proplylaxis with treatment of mild/ moderate chronic asthma 2–5 y => 4 mg/dose o.d. in the evening orally 6–14 y => 5 mg/dose >15 y => 10 mg od

DRUG THERAPY IN SEIZURES

	Simple febrile seizures	Atypical febrile seizures
Episode	1/day	>1/day
Seizure type	GTCS (or) Tonic clonic	Usually partial or complex partial
Duration	< 15 minutes	> 15 minutes
Age group	6 months – 60 months	May come < 6 months and > 60 months
Focal Neurological Defects	No	Yes
Prognosis	Good	Not to miss if being treated for seizure disorder (or) acute CNS infection (or) febrile status epilepticus

TREATMENT FOR FEBRILE SEIZURES

1. Reduce fever
2. Diazepam: Oral: 0.33 mg/kg/dose 8 hrly
   Rectal: 0.5 mg/kg/dose
3. Clobazam: 0.25–1 mg/kg/day b.d. or t.d.s.
4. Treat iron-deficiency anemia

Initial Drugs

1.	**Inj. Lorazepam**	0.05 mg–0.1 mg/kg IV (OR)
	Inj. Midazolam	0.15 – 0.2 mg/kg IV or IM (OR)
	Inj. Diazepam	0.2 mg – 0.5 mg/kg IV

Oral Anti-Seizure Drugs (Not Status Epilepticus)

1.	**Phenobarbitone**	Oral: 3–5 mg/kg/day **IV loading dose: 10–20 mg/kg over 20 minutes**
2.	**Phenytoin**	Oral: 5 mg/kg/day **IV loading dose: 10–20 mg/kg over 20 minutes. Dilute with normal saline**
3.	**Sodium valproate**	10 mg/kg/day to begin, increase by 5 mg/kg/week Maximum 30–40 mg/kg/day
4.	**Levetiracetam**	10 mg/kg/dose 12 hrly; increase every 2–4 weeks to max of 30 mg/kg/dose
5.	**Carbamazepine**	Mainly for partial seizures. 10 mg/kg/day b.d. or t.d.s. max up to 20 mg/kg/day

SKIN ALLERGY

Urticaria

1.	**Hydroxyzine**	1–2 mg/kg/dose 8 hrly 10 mg
2.	**Cetrizine**	2.5–5 mg/day 2–6 years 5–10 mg/day 6–12 years
3.	**Prednisolone**	1–2 mg/kg/day b.d.
	Topical	Calamine lotion application

- Not to miss Anaphylaxis, where O_2 intramuscular Adrenaline and large volume isotonic fluids are life-saving.
- Look for ENT, Dental and urosepsis if urticaria is persistent or recurrent.

CONSTIPATION

Rule out hypothyroidism and iron-deficiency anemia.

1.	**Increase fiber diet**	
2.	**Bisacodyl**	Oral and suppository 1–5 years => 5 mg > 5 years => 10 mg
3.	**Lactulose**	0.5 ml/kg/dose 12–24 hrs
4.	**Paraffin liquid**	1 ml/kg daily

APPENDICES

Emergency Medications

Medication	Dose	Maximum single dose	Route/Comment
Adrenaline 1:10,000 (0.1 mg/mL), 1:1,000 (1 mg/mL)	0.01 mg/kg or 0.1 ml/kg of 1:10000	0.5 mg	IV, IO.ETT (IM in anaphylaxis) (SC in near fatal asthma)
Atropine	0.02 mg/kg	1 mg	ETT, IV, IO
Calcium Gluconate (10%) (1 ml = 100 mg)	0.5–1 mg/kg	2 gm/dose (20 mL)	IV. IO, slowly IM
Magnesium Sulfate (50%) (500 mg/ml)	25–50 mg/kg 0.05–0.1 ml/kg	10 mL (50% soln.)	IV over 1/2 hr
Lidocaine* *(Prefer preparations without preservatives—Xylocard)	1 mg/kg	40 mg	IV, 10, ETT
Adenosine (SVT)	0.1 mg/kg (*1st dose) 0.2 mg /kg (2nd dose)	6 mg (1st dose) 12 mg (2nd dose)	IV followed rapidly by 10 ml saline flush
Amiodarone (Pulseless VF or VT-perfusing tachycardias)	5 mg/kg (Over 20–60 min.)	150 mg	IV, IO
Adrenaline 1 : 1,000 (Nebulized) Croup	0.5 mL/kg	< or = 4 yrs – 2.5 mL > 4 yrs–5 ml	Inhalation
Salbutamol (20 min. × 3)	<20 kg - 2.5 mg >20 kg- 5mg		
Activated charcoal	1 gm/kg	50 gm	NG tube or PO
Sodium bicarbonate (1 ml = 1 mEq) Used only if Ph < 6.9	1 mEq/kg Dilute 1:1 (distilled water)	N/A	IV, IO
Electric shock dose	Synchronized Cardioversion—0.5–1 J/kg (may increase to 2 J/kg if ineffective. Defibrillation–2 J/kg (1st dose), 4 J/kg (2nd and subsequent doses.)		

Inotropes, Vasopressors, inovasopressors, Inodilators and Vasodilators

Medication	Usual dose (mcg/kg/min)	Dilution in 50 ml D5W	IV infusion rate
Dopamine	5–15	30 mg/kg	1 ml/hr = 10 mcg/kg/min
Dobutamine	5–20	30 mg/kg	1 ml/hr = 10 mcg/kg/min
Epinephrine	0.05–1.0	0.3 mg/kg	1 ml/hr = 0.1 mcg/kg/min
Norepinephrine	0.05–0.5	0.3 mg/kg	1 ml/hr = 0.1 mcg/kg/min
Vasopressin	0.02–0.06 units/kg/hr	1 unit/kg in 50 ml D5	1 ml/hr = 0.02 unit/kg/hr
Milrinone	0.5–0.75	1.5 mg/kg	1 ml/hr = 0.5 mcg/kg/min
Sodium nitroprusside (SNP)	0.5–4	3 mg/kg	1 ml/hr = 1 mcg/kg/min
Nitroglycerine (NTG)	0.5–5	3 mg/kg	1 ml/hr = 1 mcg/kg/min

FLUID CALCULATIONS IN BURNS

Use the Parkland formula (below) as a guideline to estimate fluid need (note that this formula provides for replacement and losses, not maintenance fluids. So, one must add maintenance fluid requirements).

1. **First 24 hours:** Administer 4 ml/kg of crystalloid percent BSA burned, over the first 24 hours; Infuse half of total dose over the first 8 hours calculated from the time of injury and the remaining half over the next 16 hours.
2. **Second 24 hours:** Fluid requirements constitute 50% to 75% of the first day's requirements. Determine concentrations and rates by monitoring weight, serum electrolytes, urine output, nasogastric losses, etc.
3. **Consider adding colloid after 18 to 24 hours (albumin 1 g/kg/day) to maintain serum albumin > 2g/dl.**
4. **Withhold potassium-containing fluids for the first 48 hours,** since a large amount of potassium is released from damaged tissues. To manage electrolytes effectively, monitor urine electrolytes twice weekly and replace urine losses accordingly. Urine output should be maintained at ≥ 0.5 ml/kg/hour.

AIRWAY CALCULATIONS

Both cuffed and uncuffed ET tubes are acceptable for infants and children; avoid excessive cuff pressure in case of cuff ET tube.

ET SIZE

Uncuffed $= \dfrac{\text{Age (years)}}{4} + 4$

Cuffed $= \dfrac{\text{Age (years)}}{4} + 3.5$

Depth from lip (in cm)* Age (yrs) {Add 3 cm for nasotracheal tube)

$$\frac{\text{Age (years)}}{4} + 12$$

*Verify accurate placement clinically and radiologically

Airway:	Oral	Central incisors to angle of jaw
	Nasal	Nose to tragus of ear
Weight:	1-6 years (in kgs)	8 + 2 × patient's age (years)
	6-12 years	7 × age (years)- 5/2

SEDATION INFUSION

Drug	Dose
Morphine	20–80 mcg/kg/hr (1 mg/kg in 50 ml 5% Dextrose, 1 ml/hr = 20 mcg/kg/hr)
Fentanyl (Analgesic)	1–5 mcg/kg/hr
Midazolam (Sedative)	1–4 mcg/kg/min
Dexmedetomidine (Sedative)	1 mcg/kg IV over 15 min., then 0.2–0.7 mcg/kg/hr

SEDATION HOLIDAY

(Stopping sedation infusion from early morning for few hours and allowing the child to wake up).

This reduces risk of ventilator-associated pneumonia and allows better neurological assessment.

If child is agitated or uncomfortable, restart sedation.

VITAL SIGNS

Age	Respiratory rate (Min-Max)	Heart rate (Min-Max)	Systolic blood pressure (Min-Max)	Distance (CM) Mid-trachea to lip
Preemie (1–2)	30–60	90–180	50–70	8
Newborn (3–5)	30–60	90–180	50–70	8–9.5
6 MO (7)	24–40	85–170	65–106	9.5–11
1 YR (10)	20–40	80–140	72–110	11–12.5
3 YR (15)	20–30	80–130	78–114	12.5–14
6 YR (20)	18–25	70–120	80–116	14–15.5

Contd...

Contd...

8 YR (25)	18–25	70–110	84–122	17–18.5
10 YR (30)	16–20	65–110	90–130	18.5–20
12 YR (40)	14–20	60–110	94–136	20
15 YR (50)	12–20	55–100	100–142	20–21.5
18 YR (65)	12–18	50–90	104–148	20–23

EQUIPMENT

Endotracheal tube (uncuffed)	Laryngoscope blade	Suction catheter (FR)	NG tube (FR)	Foley's catheters (FR)	Chest tube (FR)
2.5–3.0	0 straight	5–6	5	5 feeding	8–10
3.0–3.5	1 straight	6	8	5 feeding	10–14
3.5–4.0	1 straight	8	8	5 feeding	12–16
4.0–4.5	2 straight	8	10	8 Foley	14–20
4.5–5.0	2 straight	8	10	10 Foley	18–22
5.0–5.5	2 straight	10	12	10 Foley	20–28
6.0–6.5	2 straight/curved	10	12	10 Foley	28–32
6.5–7.0	3 straight/curved	12	14	12 Foley	28–32
7.0 (cuff)	3 straight/curved	12	14	12 Foley	28–32
7.0–7.5 (cuff)	3 straight/curved	12	16	14 Foley	32
7.0–8.0 (cuff)	3 straight/curved	12	16	16 Foley	32